Slaying the Cancer Giant
with the
WORD OF GOD

An Autobiography of a Cancer Survivor

Rev. Dr. Diana Fields

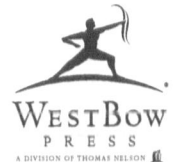

WESTBOW
PRESS
A DIVISION OF THOMAS NELSON

Unless otherwise indicated, Scripture quotations marked NLT are taken from the Holy Bible, New Living Translation, copyright 1996. Used by permission of Tyndale House Publishers, Inc., Wheaton, IL. 60189. All rights reserved.

King James Version, Zondervan Publishers, Grand Rapids, MI, Copyright 2000.

WestBow Press books may be ordered through booksellers or by contacting:

WestBow Press
A Division of Thomas Nelson
1663 Liberty Drive
Bloomington, IN 47403
www.westbowpress.com
1-(866) 928-1240

Because of the dynamic nature of the Internet, any web addresses or links contained in this book may have changed since publication and may no longer be valid. The views expressed in this work are solely those of the author and do not necessarily reflect the views of the publisher, and the publisher hereby disclaims any responsibility for them.

Any people depicted in stock imagery provided by Thinkstock are models, and such images are being used for illustrative purposes only.

Certain stock imagery © Thinkstock.

ISBN: 978-1-4497-6061-8 (sc)
ISBN: 978-1-4497-6063-2 (hc)
ISBN: 978-1-4497-6062-5 (e)

Library of Congress Control Number: 2012912993

Printed in the United States of America

WestBow Press rev. date: 12/13/2012

Contents

In Memory of My Mother and Grandmother

This book is written in memory and honor of my mother, who died of breast cancer, and my grandmother, who died of leukemia. It is a written voice for those who are also struggling and have struggled with this devastating and debilitating disease. The book speaks from a first person perspective while telling a compelling story of my own personal struggle with cancer.

I give honor to my mother and grandmother because of their heroic battles with cancer. Since I was primary caregiver for both of them, I received valuable information about the disease. Even though they struggled with different kinds of cancer, I was able to observe and learn a great deal about each. However, in this book I share my personal feelings in caring for my mother and her difficult and painful bout with the disease. I give honor to her and God that I was able to complete this book for the purpose of touching and encouraging the lives of people facing devastating situations like cancer, as well as other stressful events in life.

Through my own bout with cancer, and also through being caregiver of my mother, who succumbed to this disease, I have gleaned some important lessons that I wish to share with others. I hope that this book will encourage and inspire those who have travailed through this disease to share what they too have learned from their experiences. I encourage you to join with me in spreading the reality that women and men should pay attention to their bodies and physical warnings that might lead to something more serious than expected.

In the pages of this book there are inspirational scriptures, informational sections, and biblical stories to assist you in building faith and a personal relationship with God. Throughout this book it is hoped that my own personal faith in and relationship with God shines through to the readers. As my faith shines through, I hope that your spirit will be illuminated too.

Acknowledgments

Words cannot express the encouragement, and support that my editor, Deborah Bennie, has given me. I want to thank her for taking the time and making the effort to walk alongside me in the writing of this book. Her professionalism and expertise helped to make its contents a true testimony of the faithfulness of God. Deborah's persistence kept me focused on writing this book and continuously on task. Her gentle prodding was just enough to keep me going. I believe it was her steadfastness in wanting to complete this book with me that propelled me to finally finishing it.

Deborah challenged me when I needed challenging. She corrected me when I needed correcting and cheered me on when I needed cheering. Her quiet presence and input have been the driving forces in me, producing this final product. I want to publicly thank Deborah for all of her dedicated time and effort in helping me create this book.

The writing process has been a long journey, and I have agonized over whether this book is worth the paper it is written on. Now that it is complete, I am convinced that it will be a blessing to many people. The personal struggle I had while writing this book affirms and confirms for me that it is written from the very depths of my heart in order to touch the hearts of others. The purpose of this book is to encourage people who are painfully and emotionally suffering from devastating diseases and those who are experiencing hardships in life. Trust God in all situations.

Thank you, Deborah, and may God bless you. I look forward to working with you on my next endeavor!

Introduction

One goal of this book is to share with women and men the knowledge I gained during my nine-month bout fighting breast cancer. The fact is that breast cancer can affect both women and men. So men, don't think this book is not for you. Besides the other cancers that plague men, breast cancer is occurring in men as well. Monthly breast self-examinations in women and men are essential for early detection.

When a nurse first asked my husband if he performs self-examinations on his breasts, he burst out in laughter—until he realized she was serious. She shared with him that men can have breast cancer too, though it is publicized very little. He was shocked to say the least. Now I believe he realizes the importance of performing monthly breast examinations. Breast cancer is no laughing matter. Breast cancer does kill thousands of people each year. To women who are reading this book, make sure you pass this information on to the males in your life.

I have written this book in an attempt to inform women *and* men of the importance of acquiring information on health issues that can seriously affect their lives. We still must realize that all the facts about cancer have not yet been discovered, otherwise there would be a breast cancer cure! So knowing the facts that are available can help you to be a more informed and prepared person.

Facts now indicate that if there is a strong breast cancer history in a family, whether on the mother's side or the father's side, there is a greater chance that a male *or* female in that family will have breast cancer. Breast cancer is destructive, debilitating, in many instances painful, and for some people a killer. Knowing your family health history is an excellent way to begin educating yourselves about your health risks. I encourage you to take the time to research your family health issues and learn the possibilities that could affect you. The more information you learn about this disease, the better equipped you are to perform preventive measures. Don't wait to find out you have some serious illnesses in your family history by being stricken with one! For those of you who find yourself hearing the words, "You have cancer," knowledge *is* power.

Through this book, I am encouraging people to get healthy. With these words, I want to remind you of how important life is and to encourage you to live it to the fullest. In order to live life to the fullest, we must make wise, thoughtful decisions that will enhance the quality of our lives. Things like self-neglect, worry, mental depression, lack of faith, complacency, and lack of knowledge can all lead to failing health, as well as a failing life journey. When you have your physical health and your mental well-being, you have everything.

Let this book be a wake-up call to those of you who don't think cancer or any other sickness can happen to you. Cancer is no respecter of persons. It strikes the young as well as the old. Sometimes it's hereditary, sometimes there is no known explanation for its occurrence, and sometimes it results from poor lifestyle choices. You and only you are the one who can change your situations and circumstances, along with the help of God. Stop right now and think about how your health can be made better by changing some of the unhealthy choices you practice. Is there something you could do better or something you should give up doing? Think and be honest with yourself!

Is there something you have been struggling with that you would like to change? If you can think of something that you would like to rid yourself of, just stop right now and ask God to help you to help yourself. Through this book, I want to bring you to the point of at least thinking about the situations and circumstances that are causing you spiritual, emotional, mental, and physical pain. Then I want to help you to understand that you can lift these things up to God in prayer, knowing that you can trust God to resolve or remove these things from your life forever.

The Autobiography Begins:
Unexpected Life Challenges

There comes a time in every individual's life when an unexpected challenge is placed in his or her path. During these times, it really feels like someone deliberately pitched you a curve ball. For the purpose of this book, I will refer to these times as *curve-of-life* experiences. If you know anything about baseball, you know that a fast curve ball can throw a batter off balance. Likewise, a curve-of-life experience causes you to swerve off the ordinary progression of life. At these crucial times, you find out who you are as a person, and your faith in God is tested. If you live long enough, you will have such an experience in your life journey. To live your life believing that every day will be free of problems and disappointments is to live life unrealistically. My faith and trust in God, my internal will, and my personal stamina were all tested. Yes, life threw me one of those unexpected curves. It was at a time when I was making good health decisions. I was exercising four to five times a week, and I was eating healthy foods. I felt better than I had for years, and I was very active.

I had set a goal to complete the Mother's Day breast cancer 3K walk in downtown Chicago. I had been walking five miles a day and felt that I was in tip-top condition. I knew I could do it! The idea to participate in the event had entered my mind many times before. However, I had never made any effort to register and participate. This time I was determined to follow through, and I did. I succeeded in getting the support of numerous financial donors. Everything was set, and I was ready to go! Mentally, I was happy. Emotionally, I was strong. Spiritually, I was alive. You could really say the world was my oyster!

The Breast Cancer Y-Me Mother's Day Walk

*T*he Y-Me 3K Breast Cancer Walk is held in May on Mother's Day. It was a commitment I felt would really honor my mother, who died of breast cancer in January 1986. I felt prepared for the task that day. I walked with my daughter-in-law and her family, so it made the day a very pleasant one filled with laughter and fun. Because there was such a large crowd, numbering in the thousands, it took the five of us approximately an hour and fifty minutes to complete the walk. And then we went our separate ways.

After the walk, I felt a sense of accomplishment, knowing I had finally put my words into action. I had no doubt that this was the time that God wanted me to do this. When I reflect back over the years that had passed, when I was unable or unwilling to make the effort, I can't really say why it took me so long. I believe God already knew that the year 2006 was the perfect year to stop the procrastination! God always has that perfect timing that lets us know He knows what He is doing and why. In the life of a Christian, it's called *the fullness of time*. You'll soon see why this was the fullness of time for me! It was time for the talk to end with action.

As life and time would have it, events following that wonderful day quickly turned for the worse. My diagnosis of breast cancer came just two weeks after I had completed the walk. I cannot describe the shock of this devastating news. This news would begin my nine-month journey and bout with an awful, life-threatening, and debilitating disease. Yes, I was thrown this unexpected curve-of-life experience! You talk about fate; what a bummer! It was through God's grace that I was able to endure a very difficult, debilitating, and overwhelming time in my life. With that said, I began to watch for and recognize the hand of God in this journey. I clung to the Bible's truths of His faithfulness and loving kindness throughout the entire experience. It was these truths that helped me to get through the whole ordeal.

A Telephone Conversation that Changed My Life

The unsettling words I was to receive that would change my life came by way of the telephone. I heard the doctor on the phone saying, "Mrs. Fields, you have a malignant breast tumor. You have breast cancer." To my own amazement, I received the words calmly. In fact, I was so calm the doctor on the other end of the phone asked me if I understood the implications of this news. I calmly told him, "Yes." Thus, I stood motionless, dazed, yet in control.

My mind was weighing the gravity of the news. Inside my head, I could hear the words, "Diana, you have breast cancer!" My heart was pounding a beat every millisecond, but my mind, struggling to stay in control, was asking, "Is this going to be the end for you, or will you be able to press on toward victory over your situation and take control of your medical path?" My mind and my heart told me that I had to keep pressing forward just because of who God is in my life. I had always proclaimed Him as Jehovah Jireh, *the Lord my provider*, and now I would be proclaiming Him even more as Jehovah Rapha, *the Lord that healeth*.

At that very moment, I made the decision to press on with the help of God through much prayer. I was convinced that effectual, fervent prayer, excellent doctors, medical breakthroughs, along with my strong faith in God, would get me through this ordeal. I understood that it was going to be a difficult journey and the road would be rough, but I couldn't allow myself to forget that "with God all things are possible" (Matthew 19:26). So I began to cast my cares upon the Lord and let Him direct my path.

I have learned a few things in my sixty-six years of life, and one important thing that I have learned for certain is that God never takes you to something difficult that He won't go through with you. Yes, He was right there with me every rough step of the way. These unexpected curves in life are tests of faith and learning experiences to make you the person God intended you to be. Without these tests there would be no testimonies! I knew then that this was to be one of my tests.

During that phone call, my husband stood nearby, watching the reaction on my face and discerning that something was wrong; he quickly embraced me to help me keep my balance. I simply stood looking dazed and feeling weak in the knees. I did understand all too well the implications, because some twenty-plus years before, I had seen my mother battle the breast cancer giant. Although I knew there was a real possibility that I might someday get cancer, I had never spoken the possibility aloud.

Let me explain how this telephone conversation came about. Shortly after I had completed the 3K walk for breast cancer, I was notified by my local hospital that it was time for my yearly mammography. So I scheduled an appointment to have it done. The appointment began as a normal and uneventful screening. Once the screening was completed, the technician took the screening a step further and asked me if I had any complaints or problems concerning my breasts.

That question changed that routine annual screening into an unexpected event. I actually did have some concerns, and when I conveyed them to the technician, I ended up having two mammographies done that day. The second mammography was a more diagnostic screening than the first. I went in with confidence that all would be well. I wasn't expecting the screening to have changed from the year before. However, since we don't know what's going to happen from one minute to the next, we are sometimes thrown a curve in life that catches us totally off guard. This appointment was one of those moments. As a result of the second test I took that day, I found out that I had breast cancer. I was very glad that I had taken the time and the initiative years earlier to begin mammography screening. I believe this saved my life!

Keeping Track of Your Health

Keeping track of my physical health was something I believed in doing. Since cancer was in my family history, I started very early having the yearly screenings. I chose to keep a close track of what was happening with me. For me there was no other option. Cancer had already struck twice in my family. My mom died of breast cancer, and later my maternal grandmother died of leukemia. Needless to say, I certainly understood the importance of my diligence after I was diagnosed with cancer. I don't want to imagine what my prognosis might have been if I had not begun this process years before. So now, I make the plea to all women who are too afraid to make that first phone call to use me as an example. As scary as it might seem, you couldn't make a more important call as the one that might save your life. Schedule your mammogram. Start to keep track of your health. It is imperative that you do.

Cancer is on the rise not only in the African American community, but in all communities. I sat with Asians, Latinos, Jews, Hindus, and many other ethnicities as I underwent both chemotherapy and radiation treatments. There were young women, middle-aged women, and older women all taking treatments. Even though we were from very different backgrounds, we all had one thing in common—we all had cancer!

As I said earlier, cancer is no respecter of persons. It strikes the poor, the rich, the famous, and those little known. Everyone is at risk for having this devastating disease. Breast cancer is not the only cancer that is wreaking havoc in our world, but many different types of cancers are appearing. For example, I had never even heard of muscle cancer, but it does exist. Eye cancer, cancer of the tongue, skin cancer, lung cancer, prostate cancer, colon cancer, stomach cancer, and many others are showing up in all age groups and ethnic groups.

Why wouldn't a person want to get a yearly physical so that any irregularities can be detected and treated early? I'm writing this book for those men and women who believe that regular physical checkups are unnecessary, or that you can't fit them into your busy schedule, or that cancer won't happen to you. Time is ticking away, and there's no guarantee that any of us will escape serious illness. There are so many different things happening with our foods and in our world that could affect your health that I would think that everyone would want to keep track of these things and start a preventive health course.

So what are you waiting for? Are you waiting for some illness to bring you down, or are you just naive in thinking that you will never get sick? There are people who are sick with devastating illnesses who lived a healthy lifestyle their entire lives, but still they are sick. Then there are those who never grace the doors of a doctor's office who are walking around completely well. Now it's a 50/50 chance of going either way. However, you as an intelligent individual can help your physical condition along in a positive manner by monitoring your personal health and by seeing your doctor on a regular basis. Don't let fear keep you from having yourself checked out. The only thing you must fear is fear itself. Fear can paralyze you to the point of inactivity. Overcome fear with self-determination. Check yourself before you wreck yourself and your life!

We know that fear is not from God. Study God's Word so that you will know for yourself what God says he'll do for you in sickness, in your daily living, and in unexpected life situations. A daily dose of His Word will help keep your spiritual and emotional life strong, but through a professional medical team you can help to keep your physical body strong as well.

Even though we know that God is the Great Physician, we also know that he uses trained medical professionals to treat our ailments and to keep our bodies well. Life is too precious to take unnecessary chances with our health. A yearly checkup is really not a lot to demand of yourself when you consider the consequences of neglecting to do so. Tell yourself that it takes one checkup to save your life! I am a prime example of that. Remind yourself that being proactive about taking care of your body is necessary in order to maintain good health.

The Power and Effect of Words When Going through Cancer

*W*ords and thoughts have power. That's why I encourage you to think seriously and realistically, yet positively, about the state of your health. Words and thoughts can inform, misinform, direct, and misdirect the path of your life decisions. It is absolutely necessary that we think positively about how we have the power to affect our mental and physical health. The Bible says that "life and death are in the power of the tongue" (Proverbs 18:21 AKJV). Words can destroy. Words can tear down, or words can build up and restore. We take words into our minds, whether positive or negative; therefore, the mind is a powerful influence on how we see ourselves and how we respond to different situations and circumstances. The words contained in our thinking suggest ways of acting and responding in different situations. However, we do have control over what we think and speak. We have the choice whether or not to think or speak certain thoughts.

In the book of Ephesians, chapter 6 tells us we must put on the full armor of God each and every day, and 1 Thessalonians 5:17 says we are also to pray without ceasing. In other words, we must always pray, and establish it in our minds that we must strive to live victoriously, so that we can declare the works of God in our own lives and in the lives of others! We must remember those Scriptures we have learned from the Bible that help to keep our minds at peace. We do need a mind of peace when we're going through times of struggle and testing. Speak positive thoughts and positive words to yourself as you journey through cancer.

You must find things to do that keep your mind occupied in a positive way. There is an old saying that "an idle mind is the Devil's workshop!" Slay that cancer giant by conquering destructive, defeating thoughts with the weapon of God's Word. Say, "I shall not die, but live, and declare the works of the Lord!" (Psalms 118:17 KJV). Slay unproductive thoughts concerning your healing with positive affirming words that strengthen you. Memorize Bible verses that help to empower you for your situation. Don't allow negative, unproductive thoughts to rob you of your peace as you face adversity. Start by declaring that "I can do all things through Christ which strengtheneth me" (Philippians 4:13 KJV).

There is something about the Word of God that helps to defeat the tricks of the enemy. Satan, our enemy, delights in our failing these challenges of life. For those of you who don't believe that Satan exists, you're right where he wants you to be. Don't stay in denial of the fact that he does exist in the spiritual realm. If he can keep you ignorant in the spiritual realm, he can continue to wreak havoc in your life. However, the Holy Bible and all its authority will negate all of the power that Satan tries to exert over you and your life. It is true that he does go to and fro throughout the earth seeking whom he may devour (1 Peter 5:8 KJV).

How I Got Myself and My Mind Together

 *M*any problems we face start from thoughts or beliefs warring in our minds. When I received my results by telephone, my mind at that particular moment said to me, "Diana, how are you going to react to this news? Are you going to go into an uncontrollable rage, or are you going to trust in God and draw upon your faith, as you tell others to do in times of great struggle?" And guess what, Satan was right there whispering to my mind, "I got you now!" As a Christian, I had to remember that Satan (our enemy) has no power in my life.

I reminded myself that Satan has already been defeated by the blood of Jesus on the cross of Calvary. Sometimes the enemy will come in like a flood, but God will raise up a standard against him! That is a believer's promise, hope, and comfort. Sickness, disease, trouble, pain, and mental agony will have to cease when we allow God to be in control. Allow God to control your mind and thoughts. We do this through daily reading of the Word of God, which is the Holy Bible. Your thoughts can do a great deal of damage to your healing process. Is allowing your mind and thoughts to control you (rather than allowing God to control *them*) worth losing out on your physical, spiritual, and emotional health? I don't think so.

The minute I decided to let God keep me and my mind at peace was a critical juncture in my journey. I know now that God was allowing me to use my free will to decide whether I would trust Him throughout this ordeal or fall to defeat by allowing the adversary to place my mind in bondage to fear. Fear is not from God, and if something is not from God, then it has to be from the evil one, Satan. I deliberately took a stand to trust God and activate my faith in Him! I put fear behind me and never entertained it again!

I had to remind myself that Isaiah 53:4-5 (NIV) says, "Surely he took up our infirmities and carried our sorrows, yet we considered him stricken by God, smitten by him; and afflicted. But he was pierced for our transgressions, he was crushed for our iniquities, the punishment that brought us peace was upon him, and by his wounds we are healed." "For God has not given us a spirit of fear and timidity, but of power, love, and self-discipline" (2 Timothy 1:7 NLT). This holds true for all believers. Therefore, I had to remember to keep my mind focused on Jesus, for He said, "Thou wilt keep him in perfect peace whose mind is stayed on thee, because he trusteth in thee" (Isaiah. 26:3 KJV).

As I spoke the Word of God or read the Word of God, as I travailed through my bout with cancer, I found victory over the enemy! Satan wants to control your mind. If he knows he has your mind, he will begin to work on your thoughts. He wants to destroy every positive thought you have that keeps you focused on God. He wants to take those positive thoughts and turn them into negative thoughts concerning God so that you will begin to distrust and doubt the love, faithfulness, authority, and the power of God.

We must learn to do what the Scriptures say and bring into captivity every negative thought to the obedience of Christ (see 2 Corinthians 10:5b). This means that we should be vigilant about bringing into captivity every thought that does not line up with God's Word. Fearful, self-defeating thoughts and those that lack trust in God are to be brought in line with the Word of God. When you're not sure of your faith, trust in God and ask Him to become the head of your life and be your Lord and Savior. Don't give Satan the opportunity to control your body, mind, and soul. Salvation is the believer's assurance of victory over all sin and death! Salvation saves us from the ultimate eternal fire of damnation. The Bible says, "Whoever calls on the name of the Lord shall be saved (Acts 2:21 KJV).

Satan wants you to think about negative results and prognoses. He will try to overshadow you with fear. Believe in God's Word (the Holy Bible), hold firmly to its promises, and you will slay the Devil and all of his schemes. You must have a strong faith and trust that God will do what He says He will do in His Word. Ultimately, it is God's *will* that will be done!

The Scripture that I held on to throughout my bout with cancer was Deuteronomy 31:8, which states, "The Lord himself goes before you and will be with you; he will never leave you, nor forsake you. Do not be afraid; do not be discouraged" (NIV). This should bring someone going through a devastating disease like cancer or any other difficult situation a great deal of comfort, because we know that God's Word is true and will not return to Him void. It accomplishes what He sends it out to do.

I carried that Scripture many times into chemotherapy and radiation treatments. The Word of God was never far from me. I quoted the Scriptures that I knew and found others in the Bible that encouraged me. God, His Word, and I fought the good fight of faith. I was able to gain strength by reading the Bible which helped me overcome disturbing things about various procedures, therapies, diagnoses, and prognoses. For this I am grateful!

Make up in your mind that with the help of God you're going to overcome your situation. This mindset does, however, require courage and determination. You must walk by faith from the very beginning of your journey with cancer or whatever difficult situation you face. When you do this, God blesses your faith while His Word reminds you not to fear. Press forward with determination and courage in spite of the fear you may have, but keep your mind and spirit on the goal of making it through.

It is okay to feel the fear, but *staying* in fear weakens your desire to fight on. Don't get stuck in fear; feel it, acknowledge it, and move on. When you stay in fear, your faith can't work at its maximum, if at all! Hebrews 11:6 says, "But without faith it's impossible to please God; for he that cometh to God must believe that He is, and that He is a rewarder of them that diligently seek Him" (KJV). Remember fear is the opposite of faith!

Don't try to understand or analyze why you are where you are or why you're going through what you are experiencing. Just begin to place all your faith in God because He is gracious, loving, and faithful to see you through. At some point in your journey you must decide to replace fear with faith in God. If you don't have a strong faith or any faith in God when you start your journey, whatever the journey might be, you *will* have faith when you finish your journey! Please trust me when I tell you this.

Fighting the challenging issues of life without faith in God makes your journey more difficult and definitely more challenging. People who have faith in God have learned that He is a transforming God who is able to change every situation, no matter how dismal or difficult it may seem. Thus, He has the ability to transform your fear into faith.

Medical studies now show that people who have serious illnesses like cancer and diabetes and believe in God (a higher power) tend to recover from their illnesses better than people who do not believe in a higher power. Can you believe enough in God, for this moment, to keep your hand in the hand of the One who is able to keep you? I did! Believe the doxology that says, "He is able to keep you from falling!" (Jude 24 NIV). He did keep me from falling! Many times I felt as though I wasn't going to make it, but God kept me in those difficult times, and he'll do the same for you.

Choosing the Right Health Care Staff

*Y*ou must find the place where the staff cares about your mental *and* physical health. Find the place that makes you feel like you are the most important person in the world. Make sure you get the care you deserve, no matter how difficult the diagnosis. Choose a place where age doesn't make a difference! Pray and ask God to show you where you should go. Do some research to find the right place for you. Finding the right place for your treatments is a big part of how you will feel about your success in your healing process.

I went for a consultation with the surgeon that my primary doctor recommended. I discerned him to be a very caring and honest person whom I immediately respected. His manner was relaxing, informational, and professional. I left his office feeling that he had given me his best recommendation concerning surgery. He said that he would be very willing to perform the surgery. I told him I liked his professionalism and honesty, but wanted to get a second opinion.

The second doctor told me pretty much the same as the first doctor—except the first doctor left me with the belief that a mastectomy was the best option, whereas the second doctor felt that a lumpectomy was the best treatment. The difference was that the first doctor implied that I should have my breast totally removed, and the second doctor recommended I only have the tumor removed, thus keeping my breast. However, I found that the prognosis with either of the surgeries remained the same—each surgery was expected to extend my life a number of years.

Since I had two different opinions for treatment, I felt I definitely needed a third opinion. My concern with the first two doctors was that they both worked for the same hospital and they gave me two different treatment recommendations. While I considered these two options, my neighbor came up with an idea that I really liked. She had some experience with the University of Chicago Hospital in the treatment of a medical problem with her daughter and suggested that I go there for my third opinion. She felt her daughter had received excellent care during her treatment. She gave me the name of a doctor to call to schedule an appointment for a third opinion there.

After talking by phone to a person in the breast cancer center, I was advised to gather all of my medical records as soon as I could and bring them to the center. I immediately got all of my records from the previous hospital and promptly scheduled an appointment to take them to the University of Chicago's cancer center. Surprisingly, they told me to come in the next day! I met with a staff of doctors and I left feeling that their cancer program was the best option for me. They also felt that a lumpectomy would be the route to take.

The Visit to the Breast Cancer Center

I liked the way I was treated and the professionalism of the staff when I arrived at the University of Chicago Hospital. I felt God had a hand in orchestrating this appointment! They used a medical team approach there. The idea of a team working on my case rather than an individual appealed to me. The team approach really inspired me to seriously consider the University of Chicago for my treatment

I became highly motivated and just about persuaded when I read that the University of Chicago was a top-rated cancer treatment hospital. It was ironic how that information appeared in a magazine I happened to have been reading. It was a sure confirmation to me that God had me on the right track. I knew it was God letting me know that the University of Chicago was the place I was to be treated. I didn't waste any time after that proceeding with my treatment. As the old saying goes, "The rest is history!"

Oops, a Misdiagnosed Patient!

My primary doctor, who had missed my two tumors after three examinations, wasn't too pleased with my decision to get a second and third opinion. After he discovered that I had taken my situation into my own hands (through the guidance of the Holy Spirit), he didn't have any more to say or to do with me from that time on! I had written him off after he misdiagnosed my condition during three office visits with the same complaint. His attitude left me very disheartened and angry. In fact, the very last conversation I had with him was when he left me with these words, "You need to hurry and get the situation taken care of, because the *thing* you have in your breast can be cured!"

I was taken aback to say the least. I couldn't get past the words "The *thing* you have in your breast." After that I knew I had made the right decision. His general attitude, along with his diagnosis, almost caused me to walk around with two malignant tumors for another year. He never showed any real concern for my complaints. He had no interest in further testing and he explained the result of my mammography as fibroid cystic disease and muscle strain. It seemed that the thought of sending me for additional tests never entered his mind. That's why you must continue to probe and to try to find out what really is going on in your body when you feel that something is not right. This is not a put-down on doctors, but sometimes they fall down on follow-up and follow-through! Remember what I said about how words can affect you!

By the way, I had taken my yearly mammography screening, which turned out to be negative, but because I had a technician who took some time to ask me about my breast, I was able to tell her how I felt, so she did a more in-depth screening. I also told her that I felt a lump in my breast, which my doctor had examined and said was not a lump, but a benign cyst. After this discussion the technician asked if she could examine the lump, and I told her, "Yes." She did and agreed with me that it felt like a lump and not a cyst. At this point, she asked me if I would like a more intense mammography than the one she had already given me.

She informed me that this test would be more costly, but the results would let me know with more certainty whether or not there was something in my breast to be concerned about. I told her to go for it. The type of mammography she gave me was called a diagnostic mammography. I want to stop here and advise all the women who will be reading this book to ask your doctor for a referral for this type of mammography. It is a more in-depth examination of your breast. The normal yearly screening that doctors recommend most of the time do not always find malignant tumors. So ask your doctor for a referral to have the *diagnostic* mammography. It will cost you more, but I think you will agree that it is certainly worth it! That test result changed my diagnosis!

When going through situations like this, you must be proactive rather than reactive so that you can intelligently make crucial decisions about your health care. No one knows your body better than you. Being attuned to what is going on in your body or how your body is feeling places you in the most unique position to tell others how your body feels. I knew without a doubt something was going on in my body that was not right.

It wasn't normal for my breast to ache like a toothache at night when I would lay on it. Common sense told me something was not normal because it had never happened before. I took the aches as a sign that something was wrong. I did not confuse it with muscle tension. My breast didn't ache like muscle tension, and the other clue was that it only ached at night when I lay in certain positions on it. Not only that, but my breast ached in two places. Later a second tumor was found!

The first mammography result read negative, but the second test, the diagnostic mammography, found one tumor, while the other smaller one still went undetected. Without the diagnostic mammography I would have gone an entire year with two malignant tumors undiscovered in my breast. Early detection is the key.

Men and women, take heed to this advice because the life you save might be your own. It has been proven that when a tumor is discovered, it has already been growing at least eight years before it can actually be felt. I thank God I was able to get a technician who was concerned about how I felt. God was in the midst of all of this. I give Him the praise and honor, and I thank Him for having that technician (angel) there the day I was there. I believe it was a divine setup anyway!

After much reflection, I believe God was taking control of the whole situation, even when I decided to participate in the Y-Me Breast Cancer Walk that year. I can now say that I believe He was preparing me for the journey I would travel the following months of that year. The Y-Me Walk itself now represents, for me, God telling me then that He would be walking alongside me each and every step of the way. I felt a compulsion to participate in that cancer walk, and

I wouldn't let anything stop me. I felt such a strong prodding from God that I knew I had to do it. I thought at the time it was in honor of my mom, and it was; but it was also a foreshadowing of my own journey. I now know it was also in obedience to God and that the fullness of time had come!

The Cancer Treatment Process

The first major step of my journey was to undergo a breast biopsy. This was not an easy procedure. My breast was resistant to the doctor's attempts to clip tissue from different areas of the tumor. At every attempt the doctor's instrument failed to penetrate the tumor. This caused the doctor and the attending nurses much aggravation and frustration, while causing me much pain! It was an unpleasant experience. I tell you this not to frighten you, but to let you know that the journey that you take may become difficult right from the start. So brace yourself and be aware that this journey is rough and has many bends and curves throughout.

This excruciating experience resulted in a diagnosis of infiltrating ductal carcinoma, or abnormal cancer cells in the lining of the ducts in the breast. This type of cancer is also called intraductal carcinoma. It really is hard to find anything good to say about cancer, but when this type of cancer is caught early, it's possible that the abnormal cancer cells have not spread outside the ducts to the other tissues around the breast. This is found to be the most common form of breast cancer in women. I found that nearly one hundred percent of the women diagnosed early and treated for this kind of cancer can be cured, according to the American Cancer Society.

Types of Doctors You Will Need

The following list identifies the kinds of doctors you will need to get through the cancer treatment process. If you don't have all of them, you will definitely need to see a number of them. You will need a breast surgeon, oncologist (cancer specialist), chemotherapist to prescribe and administer chemotherapy for your individual need, a radiologist to design and administer your radiation treatments, and in special instances a plastic surgeon.

Part of your care will be given by the nurses and others who will assist the doctors. These people make all the difference in the world because they can build your spirit or kill your spirit. These people should be positive and accommodating and able to help build you up mentally and spiritually.

There were times, however, during my therapy that I felt personally violated and that my personal space was invaded because of the many different hands that had to examine me. Even though I knew that the examinations were necessary, I couldn't help but to wish it to be over. Many young interns approached me with a look of embarrassment that seemed to say, "I know this can't be easy for you, with all of these strange people parading in and out of your examining room."

This is a word of caution to you reading this book. When choosing your doctor, make sure you watch how you are treated from the very first moment you arrive for consultation. The bedside manner of your doctors is very important when making a decision on who you should allow to treat you. Aloof, uninterested doctors or doctors who would rush you through the consultation process are not worth considering. Use your discernment and choose your health care staff with God's help, lots of prayer, and your gut feelings. No one knows your body like you do. No one knows what you're looking for or what you need except you and God.

You will find that there is a great deal of pressure on you as you listen and try to understand the different reports that the doctors will give you. Remember to keep the faith and know where your strength lies. Just hold on to the fact that "they that wait upon the Lord shall renew their strength" (Isaiah 40:31 KJV). There is truly strength in God's Word, which is your sword. Carry a copy of God's Word with you wherever you go, so when time permits you can feed your spiritual body with doses of Scripture. Memorize those scriptures that speak to you directly about your situation. This is how you build yourself up for battle. Even though the fight is not yours, but the Lord's, preparation will help you to be emotionally in control, mentally alert, and physically empowered.

Allow the Holy Spirit, who is your Helper, Guide, Counselor, Teacher, Comforter, and the One who will lead you into all truths about every situation, to lead you in your decision making. Don't make your selection too quickly or too haphazardly. Rely on God to keep your mind clear and free from fear and cloudy thinking. Try to stay in your right mind throughout your whole ordeal. Calm, clear, intelligent thinking is a must if you want to slay the cancer giant! Listen to your loved ones and friends who really care about you, but don't let people upset you or rush you into making decisions. Take your time, pray, think, and pray some more—really talk to God about each decision. Listen to Him, then make your decision.

My Treatment and Therapy Process

My treatment consisted of two separate surgeries. The first was performed in June, and that surgery removed a malignant tumor. A biopsy of tissue removed during that surgery revealed a second malignancy. Another surgery was done in September to remove a smaller tumor. The two surgeries took a toll on me, but complete healing from the surgeries did finally come. Not until I had healed completely from the surgeries was I able to begin chemotherapy! Chemotherapy seemed a long time coming. I found myself becoming very edgy waiting to begin chemotherapy. Waiting is not easy when you know you have a rough road ahead. I had been educated on the effects that chemotherapy had on most people. I wasn't going to pretend that it was going to be a breeze. I didn't relish the thought of losing all of my hair or having my hands, nails, tongue, and feet turn black!

Once it was started, my therapy consisted of four cycles of chemotherapy (of two weeks each) and finally thirty-three radiation treatments (six weeks, every day except the weekends). The entire therapy process was one that weakened me and made me feel tired and weary. Sometimes I could barely make it home to get in my reclining easy chair before I collapsed. There I would sit all the rest of the day, and sometimes for two or three days due to a lack of energy.

My poor husband had to do everything. He waited on me hand and foot. I am very appreciative of him for his support in caring for me and in many instances going with me for my treatment. The energy depletion and the nausea were the major side effects I had from the chemotherapy segment of the treatment. I did not experience any pain from the treatment. To say I was nauseous is not really giving the situation the gravity it deserves. Nausea after the chemotherapy was not as bad as I imagined it would be, but ugly nonetheless. Even with the anti-nausea medication, I still felt queasy.

My chemotherapy consisted of direct intravenous applications. The process is known as PUSH, which means that I did not receive my therapy through an IV port, but it was pushed directly into my veins with a needle. I liked the swiftness of my treatments and not having to sit with the IV needle in my arm for several hours. This chemotherapy treatment lasted eight weeks. One week I would have a treatment, and the next week I would rest to get ready for treatment the following week. By the time I felt like my energy was returning, it was time to go back for another treatment! That's the after effect of chemotherapy. You are totally depleted of your energy. The day of the treatment I felt just fine. In fact, on a number of occasions I actually went shopping or to a restaurant to eat afterward. The next day (it had to be exactly 24 hours later) I returned for a follow-up injection. This helped to boost the reproduction of the white blood cells. I found that this shot affected me worse than the chemotherapy. It depleted my energy entirely. Around day three the nausea set in. Even though I took anti-nausea medication, it did not completely rid me of the queasiness.

My radiation therapy, on the other hand had a more cumulative effect on my energy level. The early weeks of treatment seemed easy enough. Even though I went for radiation five days a week, there were no outward effects of the treatment early on. But, as the weeks went on, I began to feel a serious debilitating effect on my energy level. I knew that the radiation was wreaking havoc on my organs, and then my body gave way to complete exhaustion.

When the Mind and the Body Don't Agree!

Sometimes your mind will tell you that you can run to the store, clean the house, and do the laundry, but your body will not even respond to getting you up from the sofa! In other words, your body is saying, "No, I cannot and will not move," while your mind is racing to do a million and one things. Yes, I personally know that feeling. It was a very humbling experience for me while I was going through my bout with cancer. Throughout the journey, my husband, my best friend, and other friends had to take me for my hospital visits, clean my house, even shop at the store and sometimes bring my husband and me dinner. Let me tell you it's alright to let people do the things you mentally and physically are not able to do while you are going through your journey of illness.

I wanted to do all of these things for myself! Mentally, I felt I could do all of these things if I could just get out of my reclining chair! Physically, I couldn't muster up the energy to even lift my hand. The mind and the body presented two different realities on what I was able to do. So, just as the young people say, you have to learn to "take a chill pill" and allow other people to help you. Don't be too proud to ask for assistance. If friends and family volunteer to help you during your cancer journey, then they will be happy to do what they can to make your ordeal a little less stressful. They will help you during your test to help you get to your testimony. And in many instances they will be there to see you when you begin your ministry. Yes, your test does become your testimony, and your testimony will somehow become your ministry and a reason for living.

A Real Test of Faith When the Going Gets Rough

My real fight began with the therapies. It was a fight for my physical, mental, and spiritual well-being and my life. It was a fierce fight with the cancer giant because the therapies depleted me of energy to the point that I almost wanted to give up, but that was not an option for me. I was determined not to let the devastating effects of the therapies play with my mind and spirit. This is when I truly let go and let God carry me through. There was nothing I could do but pray and keep the faith at this point. I would often pray and ask God when this journey was going to be over. The thought kept coming to me that it would be over when it was over! I learned to be patient in the journey and to encourage myself by remembering that God was in the journey with me, and it would be over when He said it was over!

Remember that when the road gets rough, hard, and bumpy, and it looks like you're on the journey alone, to call upon the name of Jesus, and He will be right there with you. When it looks like things don't seem to be getting better, know that God sees and knows what you are going through, because He's there carrying you. Put all of your hope in God and watch Him transform your situation for the better. Be encouraged and learn patience, my sisters and my brothers, because God will take care of you. He will never leave you or forsake you.

Let this book be an encouragement to you when you're feeling low and worn out from being stuck with needles and from various therapies and treatments. I will be praying for all of you. I'll be praying for your complete recovery and healing. I would like to leave you with another scripture to hang on to that comes from the book of Philippians 4:6–8 AKJV: "Be careful for nothing, but in everything by prayer and supplication with thanksgiving let your requests be made known unto God. And the peace of God, which passeth all understanding, shall keep your hearts and minds through Christ Jesus. Finally, brethren, whatsoever things are true, whatsoever things are honest, whatsoever things are just, whatsoever things are pure, whatsoever things are lovely, whatsoever things are of good report; if there be any virtue, and if there be any praise, think on these things." I believe Paul is giving us a meaningful recipe for keeping our thoughts healthy and positive. The victory was mine in nine months!

On the day I made the long-awaited announcement that I had completed my treatments, I had survived eight rounds of chemotherapy and thirty-three radiation sessions! As I counted each day of my chemotherapy and radiation, I kept telling myself, "One down" and however many more to go. Chemotherapy and radiation are no joke, but if you can believe, you can receive. Control your mind by fighting off thoughts that keep you from believing you'll ever get to that day when you can say, "This is my last treatment!" Hang on to the thought that the end of this journey is coming.

In fact, I actually celebrated the completion of my chemotherapy and radiation treatments with a victory party including family and friends. There was much rejoicing, praising God, and crying! This was my way of saying, "Thank you" to all those people who walked the journey with me and cheered me on to victory. The celebration was entitled "It's Over!" I was truly a happy camper on the day I had my last treatment. My friends came over and we enjoyed the celebration that afternoon until late evening. My pastors at that time stopped by too! It was a joyous day for me. We all rejoiced in the Lord! There's nothing like a good celebration to end a faith-trying situation. God truly took me through that whole ordeal without much complaining or physical pain. I'm so glad that I knew Him and that He again was my deliverer! I can't understand how people go through difficult situations without the help of God. This truly boggles the mind.

Cancer is a disease that is frightening to most people. It is a serious and deadly disease if not caught early. However, the strides that researchers have made in treating breast cancer are such that doctors can now save lives. You just have to have enough courage to become proactive in your own physical and mental health. Although the thought of having this disease is frightening, you must remain in mental control in order to make the right decisions concerning your care.

Of course, before you make any major decision, you should always go before God in prayer to help you determine what to do. Let Him lead you in the direction you should go. This means that you should seek to hear God's voice in your situation, and then obey His voice in determining your direction. Proverbs 3:5, and 6 say to "trust in the Lord with all your heart and lean not to your own understanding, but in all your ways acknowledge Him and He will make your path straight" (NIV). Listen, obey, and then proceed; that's the path to success. God says, "I know the plans I have for you, plans to prosper you and not to harm you, plans to give you a hope and a future" (Jeremiah 29:11 NIV).

When you're trying to keep your sanity, having faith in God is not always the easiest thing to do. However, it is imperative that you hold on tightly to your faith in God when you are going through cancer or any other devastating illness. All kinds of thoughts will enter your mind to weaken your trust and faith, but remember that "God is our refuge and strength, an ever-present help in trouble" (Psalms 46:1 NIV). You must hang on to the promise that God will never leave you or forsake you as you experience the different phases of treatment.

When the journey becomes difficult, remember all of those Scriptures you memorized to keep you on the path to good health. Believe the Word of God as you say those Scriptures to yourself, while you lie on the operating table or the radiation table. As you receive the chemotherapy that will change your inner and outer body, remember the strength you can get by repeating God's Word to yourself. "For I can do everything with the help of Christ who gives me the strength I need" (Philippians 4:13 NLT).

"If God is for you, who can be against you?" (Romans 8:31 NIV). "Greater is He that is in you, than he that is in the world" (1 John 4:4 KJV). "Those who live in the shelter of the Most High will find rest in the shadow of the Almighty" (Ps. 91:1 NLT). You can find strength and determination in God's Word when you feel you have no strength. It's amazing what you'll be able to endure with God's help. He will give you supernatural power.

When the days seemed to get longer and the nights shorter, these were the times when it seemed I could hear and feel God's presence. It was during these days and nights that I heard Him tell me to stand still and see the salvation of the Lord! When I first heard this, I was totally caught off guard. This was another inspiring experience! To hear God so clearly was a new experience. I was accustomed to hearing God in a still small voice, but this time it was loud and clear! Yes, I had to realize that God was working out this situation in the spiritual realm, and all I needed to do was be still. I remembered that Jesus' death saved me from my infirmities.

If you are reading this book and you haven't asked God to come into your life to be your Savior and Lord, I am encouraging you from the depths of my heart to stop right now and say, "Lord, I repent of my sins; I want you to come into my life and be my Savior and Lord. I do believe that Jesus is the Son of God, and that He died for all of my sins. Come and live in my heart." God *will* come and live in you.

I don't know how I would have made it through my cancer treatments without knowing that I had a God I could depend on. I believe this was something I had to experience in order to understand that God can do all things. Life is under His divine direction. God is a part of everything that happens in life. I believed that God would heal me through the doctors. I was confident of this from the very beginning.

However, I can't tell you how many times my faith was tested. Hebrews 11:1 (KJV) states, "Now faith is the substance of things hoped for the evidence of things not seen." Being able to believe you're totally healed without immediate manifestation or evidence is a difficult mindset for most people. This is when your faith gets challenged. "It is impossible to please God without faith" (Hebrews 11:6 NLT). Faith is the thing that gets God moving and working on your behalf.

Journeying with My Mother through Breast Cancer

As I reflect back over my journey with my mother and her bout with cancer, I find it difficult to think about. The pleasant memories of my mother's cancer experience were right after her initial mastectomy surgery when she lived four years cancer free. Our family was filled with happiness and hope. She lived a good normal life. She worked every day and touched the lives of the people she encountered working as a currency exchange manager. She was an encouragement and brought joy to many people. She had a personality that drew people to her. She was small in stature but had a heart larger than life. She had a heart for people.

When I think back on the day when we found out her cancer had returned, the memory of it is still very painful. My mother's fight against cancer was not an easy one. With my grandmother and I being the primary caregivers, the journey in caring for my mother was also difficult for us. Caring for a person who is debilitated by cancer and watching the process that disables them to the point of emaciation is heart wrenching. This person who gave me birth, who loved me unconditionally, and had been with me all my life was now so sick that words could not describe the pain I saw her suffer. This takes a devastating toll on the caregivers. It is emotionally, mentally, psychologically, and physically draining. I can't tell you how hurtful it was to see my own mother struggle through this disease. I was in constant prayer with the Lord asking Him to heal her. However, it was ultimately God's will for her to take her rest.

The experience of being a caregiver to my own mother was an experience I will never forget. The thoughts that come with remembering bring me close to tears. The sleepless nights both my mother and I endured invade my thoughts. I remember how I would sometimes read the Bible to her because she couldn't or wouldn't go to sleep because of the pain. The suffering that I saw my mother endure was indescribable and etched within my thoughts forever. Although she suffered silently, I knew she was fighting a giant that was relentless. Her face and body could not conceal what I knew to be nothing but unadulterated pain. Yes, I had my experience with suffering as I journeyed with my mother through her cancer. It was a mental suffering that I can't even talk about to this day. It was a roller coaster of a ride. I was up when I thought my mother was improving, and I was down when the real truth of the situation grasped me. I surprise myself even now being able to write about these things.

Nevertheless, I can say with some assurance that the caregivers of the sick mentally experience the illness right along with the person who is sick, not to the extent of having the sickness but to the extent of the mental anguish. You just can't watch someone you love suffer and not be affected by it. Well, time has healed some of the unpleasant memories of caring for my mother during her illness, but it will never erase all of the memories. However, the very private and wonderful moments that I shared with my mother during her somewhat lengthy illness are memories that I will hold close to my heart forever.

There is one thing that I must say about my mother's bout with cancer that really is a testimony to the reality of God. I really saw my mother's relationship with God change in a very powerful way. I saw my mother change from a person who rarely read and studied the Bible to a person who daily and on many days, all during the day, began to read, study, and meditate on the Word of God. I witnessed a spiritual change in my mom that caused her to begin to pray, to praise God, and to build a personal relationship with God that took her to another level of being. She seemed to be preparing herself for her final journey. Her countenance also changed. You could see a peace upon her that she didn't have at the beginning of her journey. My mother had been a Christian for as long as I could remember, and yet I had never seen her seek the Lord like she did during her last days on this earth. Her faith in God became quite evident as she approached her last days. It made me understand how important it is to have that close and personal relationship with our Creator God to the point that we talk to Him all the time, knowing He does hear and answer prayers. Watching my mother became a real testimony of how we must trust and rely on God in every situation. It was a real learning experience for me when I faced cancer myself. I thank God I was able to witness the transformation in my mother's faith as she prepared for her final journey to be with the Lord. It really made a difference in how I approached my own episode with breast cancer years later.

This was twenty-six years ago, and since then tremendous strides have been made in the treatment of cancer. I thank God for the continued advances in chemotherapy and radiation treatments. With more individualized treatments of patients, cancer is being controlled and even cured in many instances. Early detection is the key. My mother waited for quite a while before she went to the doctor to ultimately be diagnosed with breast cancer. She was always afraid to go to the doctor because she had always felt that she would get cancer. It turned out to be a self-fulfilling prophesy. Because she had female relatives on her father's side who all died of breast cancer, she was always fearful. Fear does paralyze. Fear does immobilize people. That's why it's so important to focus on God in fearful and stressful situations. Only God can keep your mind and thoughts in perfect peace, and also keep you moving.

I realize now that being with my mother as she was going through her cancer was preparing me for the things I would encounter as I experienced this same devastating disease. God has brought me a mighty long way. I now sit here at my office desk writing about this horrible experience that has taken the lives of many of my relatives. I want someone who is reading this book to know that you can overcome the difficult situations and circumstances in your life when you truly trust and have the faith in God that moves mountains. I hung on to God's promises in the Bible that told me all of the things that God would do for me if I just believe.

I thank God that I am now able to look back on those days and understand the relevance they held in my life as I approached my own days with cancer. Through my mother's experience I was able to make decisions that she might not have been able to make. They were decisions that helped me to overcome and not be threatened by this disease. If there was any good that came out of the experience, this would be it. I found myself knowing how to handle bad news. I was able to make decisions in difficult situations. I stood on my faith and God's guidance for direction and allowed others to help and encourage me. My mother did not have any other support other than my grandmother, my husband, my son, her sister-in-law, and myself. That was the extent of her encouragers, and that's the way she wanted it! Of course, when my mother went on to be with the Lord, her friends, and she had many, were devastated to learn that she had kept from them the fact that she had cancer. I personally felt sorry for many of them because I could understand their grief in not being able to tell her goodbye! Later in this book I talk about going public or keeping your situation private. This decision is worthy of considerable reflection!

Ten Steps to Survival

At this point, I would like to give some solid, loving advice and suggestions for going through your bout with cancer. As I was sitting in church one Sunday, God spoke to my heart about leaving the readers of this book with some tips for getting through your ordeal. I suggest these guidelines:

Pray God's Word (The Holy Scriptures) without ceasing.

Use your discernment (to perceive or recognize; make out clearly, as defined by *Webster's New World College Dictionary*, fourth edition) in making decisions.

Constantly ask God for guidance.

Keep a journal of your journey.

Ask a close friend or family member to walk with you throughout this journey.

Let this companion be your scribe, taking notes at all office visits, for your personal use.

Use the Internet to check out all of the doctors you choose to treat you. Find out about their training, experience, education, certifications, etc.

Once you have chosen them with great care, trust in your doctors and health care professionals, but trust in God first and foremost.

If possible carry your sword (the Word of God, the Holy Bible) with you to read as you wait for various appointments.

Allow God to take control of your mind through His Word—and relax.

Cancer Support Groups

There are many cancer support groups around the city and suburbs that give assistance to cancer patients. Most hospitals can direct you to support groups in your area. Cancer support groups are eager to help you make the smoothest transition back into normal life. They offer a variety of classes and support therapies that will make your journey back to normality easier. Be sure to contact your hospital's cancer support center before your treatment ends, so you will know what that hospital offers.

Many hospitals have regular meetings, speakers, and activities to help keep you informed of opportunities offered by their cancer center. My hospital offers massage sessions and classes that help you learn how to apply your makeup and find the wig that is right for you. The American Cancer Society offers free wigs to women who have lost their hair from cancer.

Find the support group that offers you the type of assistance you need to help encourage and strengthen you as you return to an active life. Find other women who have been through the process and start your own support group of acquaintances and friends. Get together with other women just to share stories and have fun. Let women who have been through the journey help you get your mental strength back. Reach out to find other women you can call on when your mind begins to speak negative thoughts into your spirit. It is good to have a network of women that you can trust, who, when you call them, have a listening ear and are available to come and be with you. Don't try to be a superwoman or one who has so much pride you aren't willing to call even your best friend!

Hopefully, the women you call upon are praying women who can get a prayer through to God. Make sure they believe in the power of God and are sanctified women of faith. Be selective of the spirits you allow into your life. Be sure the women from whom you seek support will speak blessings of healing into your life and not bring you down by sad, sorrowful, or negative remarks. I personally want to encourage you to help yourself by studying the Bible and begin hiding God's Word in your heart. Begin to strengthen yourself spiritually, mentally, emotionally, and physically with the Word of God. The Bible is excellent nourishment for the mind, body, and soul. Do everything you can to help yourself stand strongly and courageously on your feet. Share your story of faith with other people of faith and to those who may need their faith in God increased.

Finally, realize that the ultimate *support* is your relationship with God. Thank God continuously for His faithfulness, mercy, grace, and love. Remember, it is God who knows your beginning from your ending. He is the only one who knows what the plan is for your life. So don't worry or be fearful, because God is with you every grueling step of the way! I would like to leave you with this thought taken from Philippians 4:6–9 (NLT) and written by the apostle Paul, which says,

> Don't worry about anything: instead, pray about everything. Tell God what you need, and thank him for all he has done. If you do this, you will experience God's peace, which is far more wonderful than the

human mind can understand. His peace will guard you hearts and minds as you live in Christ Jesus. And now, dear brothers and sisters, let me say one more thing as I close this letter. Fix your thoughts on what is true and honorable and right. Think about things that are pure and lovely and admirable. Think about things that are excellent and worthy of praise. Keep putting into practice all you have learned from me and saw me doing, and the God of peace will be with you.

There is an old song called "God Will Take Care of You," written by Civilla D. Martin, that came to mind as I was writing this. The writer speaks to what I know to be true. God did take care of me! Now, I am able to sit and write this book that I hope will help others slay the fear of cancer! You may be wondering why I use the words *slay* and *giant* throughout this book. Well, this is the reason why: the story I reflect upon in Scripture that describes what I actually felt like as I was going through my bout with cancer is taken from the book of I Samuel, chapter 17, the well-known story of David and Goliath. David in his youth was able to slay the frightful giant with five smooth stones. I have just given you a double number of stones you can hurl at the cancer giant. I gave you ten weapons (steps to survival), which will help you resist going down to your cancer. The number ten in Scripture represents complete perfection.

The reason David was fearless of the giant was because he knew who was on his side. He knew that by believing and trusting in God that God had perfected him to fight his battle with the giant. David had the faith to believe he would overcome his foe. His mind was focused on defeating the giant. He took off things that weighed him down. He took only the weapons that he knew he needed to be successful. He mentally worked out his plan to overcome the giant. He didn't let the size of the giant evoke fear in him. He looked the giant squarely in the eye and took aim. His aim was deadly. He defeated the dreaded giant!

Cancer may look and sound like a giant to you as you face it, but fear not, because there is One who is facing it right along with you. Look squarely at your situation and proceed to fight with trust in God. Cancer can fall just like the big giant fell when David aimed the stone at a strategic place on the giant's head. Use all the weapons I listed for you previously and watch how your fear will begin to subside—strength will motivate you to press on to victory. Don't lay down your weapon (the Bible), not for a moment! Remember Satan is just looking and waiting for his chance to bring you down! Keep him at bay and under your feet. I hope the story of David and Goliath will be a good place for you to begin to reflect on your cancer battle. Begin to read and meditate on the events in this story to see what God will say to you about the battle you are fighting with cancer.

Make a promise to yourself that you will memorize ten verses of Scripture in the Bible that will help strengthen you as you prepare yourself spiritually to resist the cancer in your body. A good place to start is Ephesians 6:10–18, which describes how you must put on the full armor of God *daily*. These verses also explain what the actual armor of God is. If you haven't read or studied your Bible ever or in a long time, right now is a good time to start. Believe that you will be victorious over this disease or whatever you are battling. I can't stress faith enough. It is this combination that will win, with the help of God. Victory can be yours!

Going through the Journey
with Ample Support

God used the cancer walk as a divine setup, as well as a divine intervention. No one can orchestrate situations and circumstances like our omniscient God. I believed that I was walking in honor of my mother, who died from breast cancer; however, I would soon find that I was also walking for myself. That was the divine setup. It was a part of His fullness of time. It was the perfect time for me to discover that I too had cancer. You can't beat God's timing!

God had already worked out the divine intervention when I was notified by the local hospital that it was time for my yearly mammography! It was right after the walk that I was notified. Could the timing be any better? God intervened and sent an angel through a technician to help me. Romans 8:28 of the *New Living Translation Bible* says, "And we know that God causes everything to work together for the good of those who love God and are called according to his purpose for them." That's divine intervention! He said in His Word He would not leave you comfortless. He truly is the Father of compassion and the God of all comfort, who comforts us in our time of trouble (2 Corinthians 1:3b–4 NIV). I felt His presence in every decision I made and in every circumstance I found myself going through in that long, nine-month journey.

Other sources of strength that helped me through my cancer bout were the support, affirmation, encouragement, and prayers of friends and relatives. People far and near who weren't my personal friends were praying for me, e-mailing me words of encouragement, and calling with words to encourage me. People I didn't even know were praying for me because the people I did know who were praying for me also placed me on their prayer lists and prayer chains with their Christian friends. I was totally shocked when I was told that some Christian churches in Africa were praying for me. This for me was another inspirational time in my life. It was a special moment to find out that so many people were praying for me!

Now, the way this came about was quite unique. It was explained to me that some of my friends belong to churches that have sister churches in Africa, and they placed my name on the prayer list there when their clergy staff was visiting. Before it was all over I had people in Liberia praying for me! People I had not personally met were sending up prayers for me! What a blessing and what an encouragement it was for me.

I was truly overwhelmed with how people and the Christian saints rallied around me and walked with me through my journey. My clergy women's organization and my church were instrumental in sending up prayers, phoning, visiting, and encouraging me to keep the faith. I will never forget any of the personal conversations I had with women and even men who had gone through some form of cancer.

All of them helped me to know and understand that because God was in the mix, I would get through my ordeal. Using His Word as my battle ax, I continued to slay the giant of cancer and hold Satan at bay so that he could not infiltrate my mind. There was truly a war going on in the spiritual realm. I felt it and knew it, so I fought it the only way I knew how, with the Word of God.

Many individuals that I told about my circumstance were Christians like me. A number of my Christian brothers did call me to share the experiences they had personally had with cancer. This was very encouraging and empowering to me. To know that even men took the time to call me to tell me they were praying for me was amazing to me. If any of those brothers are reading this book, let me say, "Thank you for taking the time to encourage a sister." This to me was another example of God's divine intervention and perfect timing.

Staying Private or Going Public

This chapter addresses how you might feel about your privacy as you are going through your cancer treatment. I have already discussed the value of family and friends as your support system as you journey through your bout with cancer. This chapter, however, discusses your personal thoughts about sharing your experience with others who are not family or close friends. While I chose to go public and let everyone I knew know that I had cancer, there are those who are not comfortable being so vulnerable. I realize that many people do not share my personal thoughts on disclosure.

When I think about my own personal situation and the choice I made to share with others that I had cancer, I still believe I made the right choice. You may ask why I say this. Well, the reason is really quite simple. I knew I would have more people praying for my recovery. Just knowing that people cared enough to take a few moments to pray for me gave me great encouragement.

This also gave me a great sense of peace. To remain silent limits your support group. For me the greater the number of people who prayed for me, the more encouraged and determined I became to press forward and fight. Their words of encouragement gave me the strength I needed to stand firm in my faith. I stop now and thank all of those who prayed consistently or played any part as I was going through the process. God bless all of you for whatever role you played in helping me get through my fight with cancer. I was able to slay the giant through my prayers and yours. Prayer really does change things. There is power in prayer. As we touched and agreed in the Spirit, the giant became a weakened foe, and I became a giant slayer. A controlled and determined mind over fear became my weapon with the help of God.

My Two Companions from Beginning to End

$\mathcal{W}$ ords can't even express the gratitude I have for my husband and my best friend, who were with me from the very first appointment and continuously present for the entire nine months journey, until I had my final radiation treatment. Words cannot express the comfort I felt with the two of them by my side as I experienced my ordeal. They were my support system that gave me the strength to go on. Just knowing that they cared and were there with me made all the difference.

I felt if they could take the time out of their schedules to be with me for encouragement and support, I could certainly take the steps I needed in order to get well. There was not one moment when I felt abandoned or alone throughout the entire journey. It was their continual concern and love that spurred me on. Even though I had great support from many others, theirs was a very different and special kind of support. Their support was support that said personally to me, "I'm with you no matter what." This kind of support is what really sustains you when you're feeling down. It is the kind of support that keeps you from having a pity party about your situation. It was their love and concern that brought me out of those moments of depression and doubt.

Other Supporters

On many occasions my pastors and the first lady of our church called with prayers and words of encouragement. I remember one instance when both pastors called me together to pray for me before I was to have surgery. I left for the hospital right after they prayed for me. Their prayers encouraged me and gave me the strength and determination to face the surgeon and the surgery that was ahead. I can hear in my head right now the old song by Ry Cooder, "Jesus is on the mainline, call Him up and tell Him what you want." It came to me as I was writing today because that's exactly what I had done throughout those very trying nine months.

He did not leave me or forsake me, as His word tells us. I felt His presence and the prayers of all the saints who were praying for me every time I faced another obstacle in the treatment process. The first time I felt prayers all around me was when I went in for my breast biopsy. I actually did feel the presence of God and the presence of prayers surrounding me while I lay on the examining table. It was an experience I had never felt before. I could feel the persistence and covering of the prayers. I knew without a doubt that prayers were being prayed for me throughout the whole process. This feeling that prayers were covering me was another inspirational experience that I will never forget.

I received numerous cards in the mail, e-mails from people in and out of state, flowers, and a number of fruit baskets from different individuals. These expressions of kindness will never be forgotten. My best friends from Maryland came to visit me twice during my therapy. This was very encouraging to me. Just the fact that they took the time to visit me meant so much. Many thanks go out to my Maryland family!

I knew that I was blessed to have so many people supporting me. However, I allowed everyone to know that I had cancer and was going through a difficult time! I knew I needed every single one of them! This might have been why so many people helped encourage me. I did not keep it a secret, like it was some great embarrassment! Some women might approach it differently. Many women decide to be more secretive about their situation, and the choice really is theirs. However, I felt that I had to tell everyone so that if there was a chance that I might help to educate or to encourage someone facing a similar situation, I would be there to spur them on. You don't know how encouraging it is to hear, "You can beat this" or "You can make it!"

The Professional Support in My Journey

esides all of this support, I had the support of the hospital, its cancer team, and its cancer support center. I received three visits from the cancer support team at University of Chicago to gather information on my support systems while I was going through my ordeal. They were overwhelmed at the support I had. They informed me that many women going through the process have no support at all. To hear this made me sad.

Words cannot express the gratitude and sincere thanks that I want to convey to my oncologist, surgeon, and radiologist. These three people saved my life and were the most professional, caring, listening individuals I had ever encountered. They were honest yet understanding of my feelings, my anxieties, and my concerns. I felt that they listened to me with sincerity of heart. My oncologist was especially attentive to my personal chemotherapy treatments, and my radiologist put me at ease at the very beginning of my radiation treatments. However, my surgeon was the person whose humility I felt on a spiritual level. He was a quiet, spirit-filled man who counseled with a soft voice and a bedside manner that would win anyone over to his side. I believe we did connect spiritually. He convinced me from the very beginning that all would be well. The ease with which he was able to get me to trust him fully from the beginning was surprising.

I felt very confident in all three of these people because of their thorough step-by-step explanations of my treatments, as well as the tremendous respect they gave me as their patient. They went out of their way to let me know that I mattered and that I would be fine after the surgeries and treatments. To this day I can say, "I have been just fine!" I made it through with the help and support of these accomplished doctors and the grace of God. I want to say, "Thank you to the entire cancer staff at the University of Chicago!" Not only did you treat me, but you supported me through your continuous efforts to eradicate the cancer from my body. My thanks and prayers go out to all of you.

A Special Tribute to My Oncologist

My oncologist was a very special lady. Her credentials are too numerous to mention. However, I will mention just one. She received the genius award for her work with breast cancer in African and African American women. I was honored to have had her working on my team of doctors. She deserves the honor, respect, and accolades that she receives because of the tremendous work that she is doing to save the lives of breast cancer patients. It is hard for me to put into words how thankful I am for this gifted woman having come into my life. She is truly a giant slayer! I want to thank her for her knowledge and her tireless efforts (and the efforts of her team) in combating this devastating disease. Through her wonderful work I am sure thousands of lives (including mine) are being saved. Thank you, *Dr. Olopade*, for sharing your gift of healing. May God bless you as you continue in your quest for knowledge in slaying breast cancer. I will pray for your continued strength and intellectual giftedness as you work to find answers and a cure for breast cancer in women and men.

Special Stories of Support and Encouragement

Let me share a true story on how the power of your prayers can move God to perform miracles in someone else's life. It has been years since these personal encounters with God answering my prayers took place. Both events were eye opening for me personally on how God still answers prayers and works miracles for you and me. The first situation was when I was asked by a family member to go and pray for a young man in his mid twenties who had been admitted into the hospital for a very simple virus. While in the hospital the young man lapsed into a coma. The doctors were only able to keep him comfortable during the time he was in the coma.

For days this young man did not awaken from his comatose state. Things didn't look good for him. A friend and I went to visit him in the hospital. The doctors and the family were at their wit's end. They had even called in the priest to perform the last rites over the young man. When I arrived, his eyes and mouth had been taped shut. He had been strapped down and it just didn't look good. Of course, I wasn't expecting to see this when I arrived, so this was another curve-in-life experience for both me and my friend. Thank goodness I had asked my friend in the ministry to go with me. I know she was just as shocked and caught off guard as I was.

I had no clue what I was going to do for this young man, but I knew I was on assignment from the family and God to pray for his life. As I stood looking at him, I remember that God spoke to me and told me to ask my friend to find in her Bible the story of Lazarus. The story of Lazarus is found in the book of John, chapter 11. You should take some time to read this story; it is very moving. However, for now I'll just tell you that Jesus called out to His dead friend to come forth from death, and His friend Lazarus did exactly that.

Well I knew standing at the bedside of that young man, with his face all taped, that God was going to do something special. My friend read the story aloud, so that the young man and I could both hear it. Then I put anointing oil on my hands and begin to pray for that young man. The power of the Holy Spirit came into that room, and when I felt that power descend on me, I laid hands on that young man's head and made the sign of the cross on his forehead.

Just like in the story of Lazarus, I told the young man to come forth. Well to my surprise his body lifted slightly up off the bed he was lying on. It was almost like he had received an electric shock, the way his body responded. This was another inspiring experience for me, and I am sure I can say that it was for my friend too! I knew then that God was healing him and he was going to be a testimony of God's miracle-working power. As he lay there after I prayed, everything appeared the same. We stayed with him for a while longer, and then we left him in the same comatose state we found him in—we thought.

My friend and I made the long ride back to our homes. We talked about the experience all the way back home. When I arrived home my husband said I had received a phone call from the family member who had asked me to go pray for the young man. I returned her call and found out the young man came out of his coma just as we got on the elevator to come home. The nurse called her (the relative) to let her know that her brother was awake and doing well! Eventually I was able to shake that young man's hand when he came to my church one Sunday to say "thank you." I told him, "No, thank God!" It was nothing that I had done but what God had done through me. The power of prayer, obedience, and faith in God can work amazing miracles. God used the two of us to minister to this young man, and through our obedience and the promptings of the Holy Spirit, a miracle took place.

The second situation was when I wrote a letter of encouragement to a couple I personally did not know. I only knew about their situation. They were both in the hospital at the same time and both of them were battling cancer. There was a plea made during one of our church services by their son (my colleague in ministry) to send cards or write letters to his parents to encourage them in their journey. Well, I did write them. I didn't write them right away because I went into prayer first, asking God to help me write something that would really be an encouragement to them. So God told me to write about my own testimony and what He had done for me. I didn't just want to send a card; I wanted the letter to be personal. I wanted them to know that I had once been in their place, being in the hospital with a serious giant-size problem also staring me in the face!

I wanted them to know that even though it had been years since my lengthy hospitalization had occurred, I still remembered how it felt when a couple I didn't know took time out to come and encourage me. They did it in the kind and caring act of a hospital visit. As it turned out, my husband had mentioned to his coworker that I was in the hospital, and since we were living in the Panama

Canal Zone at the time, none of our family was nearby. In fact, I didn't even tell my family I was in the hospital! Did I miss them? Yes, but I was just too far away from home to have them try to come and see about me, so we kept it a secret. My husband and I went through the tough ordeal without the support of family. That time I decided that we must stay private! This was a tough, but necessary decision.

Well, after the gentleman heard I was in the hospital, he went home and told his wife the circumstances. They both came and visited me, without ever having met me! I was never so glad to have two individuals truly act like true Christians! They introduced themselves and told me how they had come to find out I was in the hospital. They never even told my husband, Willie, they were coming. Through my hospital stay they were a source of encouragement and laughter. Well, the rest is history. The four of us became great friends, while the men (our husbands) served in the military in the Panama Canal Zone. When I got out of the hospital, the four of us were together most of the time! What could have turned out as a most difficult experience for me turned into a most memorable and bearable one through the kindness and concern shown to me, by two strangers, during that unpleasant curve-of-life experience.

Well, after much prayer, I finally wrote to the couple in the hospital. That letter was truly a source of blessing; it encouraged them to the point of victory! How did I know? I received a telephone call from that couple when they were back home recuperating. The couple went on to tell me how my letter affected them spiritually, mentally, and emotionally. They said they knew I understood what they were going through, and they felt it. It has been at least ten years since their journey, and my understanding is that they are both still doing well. I know one of them has had a few little setbacks, but he is still making progress and doing fine.

I didn't know until then how much power the written word could have on someone. I guess that's why I decided to write this book. Now, like then, I want to encourage you because I have been there. I want you to know that you can be a living testimony and a miracle of God. My prayer is that these stories will give you a glimpse of what God can and will do for you if you trust, call out to Him, and have faith in Him.

That experience some forty-one years ago was not only a curve of life in my journey, but a valuable learning experience as well. Again, I saw the power of prayer and how it moves God into action on the behalf of others, as well as yourself. Guess what? He is still answering the prayers of His people.

Battle of the Mind after Therapy

Once you complete the therapy process, the mental journey you experience is just as challenging. Keeping your mind off negative thoughts like not being well or not being free from cancer is a major battle. I felt fine about my treatment and very positive about my survival chances until I continually heard of women who had beat cancer earlier in their lives only to have it return again to wreak even more havoc. So I became more determined to keep my mind positive and encouraged.

There is a saying that "a mind is a terrible thing to waste." I understand the significance of this saying now. What good is it for one to waste their time thinking about what may or may not happen? Life is precious and too short for us to worry about what God has planned for us or what the future holds. Why worry about whether the cancer will or will not come back? If it does or doesn't, there is absolutely nothing we can do about it or the future. Don't get me wrong—we can eat better, exercise more, and be aware of the things we do to our bodies and put in our bodies. Worrying and refusing to do the things that will enhance our overall health does nothing but defeat a healthy existence. Remind yourself as often as necessary to act wisely and to think positively.

Health Insurance Issues

I thank God that I had adequate insurance to cover my cancer treatments. I will be ever grateful for the kind of treatment and care I received because I had a husband who made sure we had adequate insurance. I am sensitive to the fact that many people who will be reading this book may not have ample insurance or none at all, nor the means to acquire any. My only plea to you is to seek counsel from an insurance professional.

If you are reading this book and don't have any form of health insurance, but you can afford it, please take the time to purchase some. If you are reading this book and don't have funds to purchase insurance, I suggest you take a trip to the John H. Stroger Hospital (Chicago) or a hospital in your area that is funded by the local government to see what they can offer you. Some medical care is better than no medical care. I wish there was more I could tell you, but I am not knowledgeable in this area. However, I mention this so that you will begin to think about what you will do if you ever need health care services. In other words, find out what options you have for health assistance. Now that the new federal health care bill has been passed, hopefully it will help alleviate such problems.

Sometimes it seems that hospitals and doctors write you off when you don't have health care insurance. They may write you off even when you do have health care if they don't think your insurance is adequate for your needs. Don't be discouraged when this happens. Sometimes doors are closed for a reason. Maybe, just maybe, God is doing something in your situation. This is when your faith in God must prevail. Exhaust all of your options for seeking medical help and give it to God.

I know you are probably saying, "How can you make something out of nothing?" My answer to you is that you can't really change your situation, but God can. So this is the time you go to God in prayer, and then leave your situation in His capable hands. Will this test your trust and faith in God? Absolutely! So while you wait to see how God will solve your problem, pray without ceasing and study His Word daily. Find a way to get help. Don't just sit and do nothing.

Turning Our Mind and Thoughts Over to God's Keeping

*B*eing proactive about staying healthy is something we all can do. Our mental health is just as important as our physical health. If you want to have peace of mind, then you'll have to allow the working of the Holy Spirit (the Spirit of God) to engulf your mind with His peace. Keeping your mind on the things of God, on God and His Word, can restore your mind and keep you in mental peace.

God's Word can ease the doubt, fear, and the devastating effects of a mind in turmoil. Remember that a worried and tormented mind is not of God, but from the enemy, the Devil. When you have peace of mind, half of your battle is won. The Bible says that the enemy comes only to kill, steal, and destroy (John 10:10). You might ask, "What does the enemy want to destroy?" The Devil wants to destroy your joy, your faith in God, your peace, and most of all—you! Sometimes we begin to think about concerns and issues that we really need to turn over to God. He's able to carry our heavy burdens, trials, and tribulations.

The Devastation of Hair Loss and Skin Discoloration

*A*ll of my doctors had informed me of all the possible side effects that could occur before, during, and after both therapies. When the things they told me did happen, I found myself somewhat prepared but still somewhat disheartened that they were actually happening to me!

One of the most devastating aspects of cancer, especially for a female, is the day you lose your first clump of hair. I can't speak for the males, but for a female, losing your hair in handfuls is a humiliating and esteem-destroying experience. A woman's hair is her crown of glory, and when you lose one of the things that you think defines you as woman, you are devastated.

I lost my hair somewhat slowly and continuously, until finally I only had just a little fuzz left. At that point I asked my husband if he could live through the task of shaving off the rest. He did appease me by shaving off the straggly little hair that was left. I know it had to be a difficult thing for him to do, but he was very gracious and courageous about it.

The lesson I learned in this part of the journey was that when I considered the alternative, I realized that hair just wasn't that important because it would grow back. It took approximately four months before it started to grow again. Each day I checked myself in the mirror to assess the progress. It was some time before I actually saw my little gray fuzz began to show on my scalp. The day I saw some semblance of hair, I was overjoyed! I felt like a million dollars just knowing that things were getting back to normal.

During the treatment the palms of my hands, the bottom of my feet, my tongue, and my nails all turned black from the intensity of the chemotherapy within my body. This was an embarrassment to me because people noticed, even though they didn't say anything. I could see the questioning and puzzled looks on their faces! Many times I would just tell them that these were the effects of chemotherapy. I believe most of them found it to be disturbing, yet also fascinating. Their response was usually "Wow!" I took it to mean that they realized that the treatment I was being given to destroy the cancer was also having a damaging effect on healthy parts of my body. As the effects of the treatments began to leave my body, my hair began to grow and my tongue, nails, hands, and feet began to return to their normal color. Now, six years later, I still look at my clear and normal tongue, nails, hands, and feet to remember where God has brought me!

Things to Do When Your Hair Is Gone

Even though you may be as bald as an eagle, there are things you can do to make yourself appealing. There were a few things I noticed about some of the women going through the cancer process that were a little disturbing to me. I noticed that many women were putting very little effort into their appearance. I saw some arriving for therapy looking unkempt. It was quite obvious that some of these women were depressed and grieving to the point of not caring about how they looked. I found for myself that getting up every day and putting on a different outfit and makeup, and periodically getting a pedicure and manicure, helped to boost my spirit. I tried to keep my routine as normal as possible. Now, granted, some days it was quite an effort to even get out of the bed, but I wouldn't give Satan the pleasure of keeping my spirits down. I was determined to keep my normal routine. For my baldness, I bought some wigs, caps, and decorative scarves. Scarves were for days I didn't want to wear my wigs. I became very proficient in making turbans and head pieces for myself. You will be surprised at what you are able to do when necessity calls. Your God-given creativity will come out if you just allow it to.

Feeling Good about Yourself

There are wonderful scarves, hats, and wigs that will help you get past the loss of your hair. Just a little bit of effort can make a world of difference in how you feel for that day. Push yourself, stretch yourself, and motivate yourself, even when you don't feel like it. In other words, make an effort to fix yourself up on a daily basis. Get up, wash up, dress up, make up, wig up, and make each day a blessed day for yourself and others. I found that when I took my mind off my situation and started to think about helping others, I felt better. Learn early in the process that sitting around feeling sorry for yourself only makes you feel worse. Get up and do something to take your mind off yourself! Volunteer to do something to help someone else.

There are all kinds of support groups and classes offered to assist you in the journey. There are massage sessions, makeup classes, wig classes, and motivational classes available. Find something that interests you and get involved while you go through your ordeal. Write a book, learn how to do scrapbooking, work some puzzles, or organize some photos. Don't just sit and do nothing!

If you don't feel like going out, you can always study the Word of God. There really isn't anything more rewarding than becoming a student of the Bible. Make something of your time while going through cancer. Start a Bible study at home. Spend time with your family. This is a time when you can grow closer to them. It is a time when you can mend some broken relationships.

Getting Control of Yourself

I have continually stressed in this book that you must allow your mind, spirit, emotions, and thoughts to focus on God and His Word. This is how we slay the cancer giant. Our thoughts must be given over to and offered up to God for His keeping. Staying stress free is our ultimate goal in order to defeat our adversary. Satan is a master mind at interrupting and disrupting our thoughts. He seeks to invade and destroy them whenever possible. He can only succeed when our faith is weak.

Be determined to focus on what Philippians 4:6–8 tells us. It says, "Do not be anxious about anything, but in everything, by prayer and petition, with thanksgiving, present your requests to God. And the peace of God, which transcends all understanding, will guard your hearts and minds in Christ Jesus. Finally, brothers, whatever is true, whatever is noble, whatever is right, whatever is pure, whatever is lovely, whatever is admirable, if anything is excellent or praiseworthy, think about such things." (NIV) I repeat this Scripture yet again written by Paul to reemphasize its important instructions to us.

There was a Scripture which I mentioned earlier, Deuteronomy 31:8, that I read and relied upon for comfort, throughout my cancer journey. This Scripture spoke to my spirit and nourished my soul. It was truly soul food! Stop and take some time to look up this passage of Scripture so that you too can be encouraged. Throughout the Bible you can find Scriptures that talk about God's healing power and protection. These will strengthen and comfort you.

Faith Healing and Laying on of Hands

Those of us who are believers know that the Bible speaks thoroughly about the healings of Jesus. There were many instances when He spoke to the disease. In other situations He touched the individuals, and on some occasions He gave individuals special instructions to follow for their healing. He had to teach the man at Bethesda (John 5:6) that much of his healing depended upon his willingness to act (become proactive) and to acquire a new mindset (renewing of your mind).

Sometimes we must become aggressive in our own healing and recovery. This is what happened with the woman with the issue of blood in the Bible. She had to press her way through the large crowd that was following Jesus to get her healing. She believed with all her heart if she could just touch the hem of Jesus' garment, she could get well (Matthew 9:20–22). She eventually did get close enough to Jesus where she could touch the hem of His garment, and she was healed! In an instant, Jesus realized that someone had touched him, because He felt some of His virtue leave him (Mark 5:30). What did this woman know and believe about Jesus that we should know today for our healing? What made her press her way into the huge crowd just to touch the hem of Jesus' garment? When you stop to think about it, she had to be on her hands and knees to be low enough to touch His hem. It wasn't like she could stand up and reach down to touch it. No, she had to get down on all fours and crawl inside the crowd to get to him.

Sometimes we have to get down on our hands and knees with our hands stretched out to God in order for God to know that we believe that He is still a healer for us today. Like the lady with the issue of blood, we must let God know that we believe, trust, and have faith in Him to the point where we are willing to crawl to Him for our healing today!

Zacchaeus, a man who was small in stature, was determined to speak to Jesus. He climbed up in a sycamore tree and called out to Him so that he might get Jesus' attention (see Luke 19:3–6). The man who was lowered through a roof in a temple so that he could be healed by Jesus was another story illustrating how we must sometimes do extreme and unusual things to bring about our healing (see Mark 2:3–5). We must be that determined. What I personally gleaned from each of these stories is that each person had a different approach to reaching Jesus to receive their healing. But there is one thing I discern that is the same in all of these stories. What stands out most clearly to me is that they all had a basic belief that Jesus could and would heal them. What is the level of your belief at this very moment? Do you believe Jesus can change your situation?

I guess you may wonder what these stories tell you about your situation and what you are going through. The answer is simple but key to your healing and recovery. I will pose the answer to you in a series of questions. Do you believe that you can be healed of cancer or whatever you are suffering from? Do you believe that Jesus, who is God, lives today? Do you believe that He wants you to be healed today? Do you believe that through the power of the Holy Spirit you can be healed of your situation? If you believe all of these things, then you can receive your health back.

You see, all the people I mentioned in the preceding stories had faith that Jesus could heal them. They trusted and believed to the point that they all were willing to take drastic actions to receive that healing. Now some people would say that calling the saints to anoint them, pray over them, and to lay hands on them would be an extreme act of faith. However, those of us who are followers of Christ know that Jesus still heals in miraculous ways. If this was not so, the Scriptures wouldn't be filled with so many verses on how we can be healed of our infirmities. He uses ordinary men and women filled with the Holy Spirit and His anointing to lay hands on people, and they *do* recover and get well. Doctors can also be included in this group.

The healing is in the sick person's belief, trust, and faith in God. Healing lies in the belief that when God sends someone to lay hands on you, that you believe that this person is being led by God to anoint you and now lay hands on you for healing. Are you raising your eyebrows over what I just said? Well, if you have a Bible handy, turn to James 5:13a, 14–16 KJV, and let's just have a little Bible study lesson in the middle of this chapter. Let's see what the engrafted Word of God says about healing of the sick. "Is any among you afflicted? Let him pray. Is any sick among you? Let him call for the elders of the church; and let them pray over him, anointing him with oil in the name of the Lord; and the prayer of faith shall save the sick, and the Lord shall raise him up; and if he has committed sins, they shall be forgiven him."

I want to leave you with these words, "If you can believe, you can receive your healing." And your blessing is in the pressing forward to get your health back. This is what the people in the stories did to get their healing. This is how you take control of your healing and slay the cancer giant! Cancer will not seem so large to overcome and defeat when you take a stand on your position over it and not let it take control over you through your mind and through fear.

Be the brave warrior that God calls you to be and fight the good fight of faith against sickness and disease. Don't throw in your sword (the Bible) before you've even tried to fight the battle or before you've even picked it up! Now our healing may not always be in the way we want it, because God knows what's best for us. Just understand that things may turn out like we expected or wanted them to—or they may not. In any case, you must understand that God always knows why things turn out as they do, because He is still in control.

The Value of Good Diet Practices

I cannot stress enough the importance of diet and exercise in cancer prevention. Before I found out I had cancer, I had gotten my body down to my ideal weight. I was eating properly and doing the necessary things to feel healthy. I was eating balanced meals containing lots of fruits, vegetables, and meats. I watched my intake of starchy foods. I was learning how to eat a low-fat diet and cooking many of my meals myself.

I paid close attention to the portions I was eating and I was dropping the pounds. I was drinking lots of water and cutting back on soft drinks and the sugary juices. My coffee and candy consumption was greatly limited. I loved my decaffeinated coffee and my chocolate candy, but I was determined to get both under control. I rarely drank alcohol, and I even eliminated the glass of wine that I might drink once or twice a month. I have never smoked, so I felt that my body was in decent condition. I was glad I had learned how to discipline myself in eating. I was learning that moderation in eating is the main ingredient to controlling your weight.

The Bible tells the story of Daniel (or Belteshazzar), Shadrach, Meshach, and Abednego in the book of Daniel 3:8. Daniel made up his mind not to defile himself by eating the food and wine given to him by King Nebuchadnezzar. Instead, Daniel asked the guard if he would allow him and his three companions to eat only vegetables and water for ten days. This was to prove that they would be as strong eating vegetables and water as the other men who ate the daily food and wine from the king's table. The story goes on to say that after the ten days, Daniel and his companions looked healthier and better nourished than any of the other young men. We can learn something from this story. The diet that Daniel and his friends followed was a simple one containing simply vegetables and water. I believe there is a definite correlation between our health and the food we eat. Food can be our strength and nourishment, or food can be our worst enemy. Daniel's story implies to us that eating a diet composed of mostly vegetables is a healthy habit.

There are lots of reasons doctors today are telling people to eat a diet composed mostly of fruits and vegetables. We live in a society where meat is acceptable to eat with every meal. Many people neglect to eat vegetables and fruits, and fast foods are the meals of the day. It's no wonder that our health is negatively affected by the foods we consume. Obesity is a problem throughout the world. I believe that just changing your diet slightly for the good will help prevent many of the illnesses that result from unhealthy eating. I know that moderation is the key. I have learned this through my own journey with eating. Even though I don't have proper eating down to a science, I am striving to be aware of what I do put into my body. Do I always eat healthy? The answer is a resounding, "No!" However, I am making strides to improve upon what I have already learned and incorporated into my eating habits. Those of you who are reading this book might want to consider monitoring your eating habits to see what changes you need to make.

Exercise, Exercise, Exercise

Today there all kinds of activities that can motivate you to exercise. Workout centers are available for the purpose of promoting good health. Living an active and productive life enhances your general well-being. Exercise helps to alleviate many serious ailments as you grow older. With diabetes, cancer, heart problems, hypertension, obesity, stroke, and high cholesterol all on the rise, we must take charge of our activity level. I couldn't do much exercise as I went through my therapies, but before I found out I had breast cancer, I did have an exercise routine.

As I reflect upon my entire life, I can actually say that I have always been pretty active and tried to always keep up some type of exercise routine. Of course, my routines have changed through the years because of my age. Now I try with some consistency to walk at least three miles when I walk. Some days are better because I am able to walk five miles. My husband and I walk three miles in approximately forty-seven minutes. It takes us an hour and twenty minutes to walk five miles. I give you this information only to encourage you to MOVE. At age sixty-six I can say that I am fairly active and have good movement of my limbs. So you get out there and walk, run, swim, or ride your bike—do something.

Spreading the Word

We know cancer is a very destructive disease that causes a great deal of damage to the body. We also know that it takes powerful therapies to destroy its devastating effects. I am hoping that this book will help combat the negative, emotional, spiritual, and mental effects of cancer by encouraging people to seek the Word of God. I want the information in this book to be more potent than the demon of cancer. I pray that God's anointed Word will go forth with healing power and authority. I want this knowledge to become contagious so that everyone who reads it will become stronger in mind, body, and soul.

I envision people all over the nation and world slaying the cancer giant through the Word of God. My hope is that people will spend a good deal of their day praying and speaking the Word of God to themselves to overcome adversity in any situation. Cancer is our focus here, but I want people to know that God's Word can be used to combat any negative or harmful situation. The tips given earlier can be used to overcome all manner of physical or spiritual warfare. Daily doses of God's Word help to build up the spiritual man and also keep the physical man built up.

You might be thinking that this book has a lot of God talk in it, and you're absolutely right. As an ordained minister, I am writing this book to glorify God for His goodness and faithfulness in my own life. I don't apologize for my strong theological emphasis. My bout with cancer was challenging, yet empowering, because God gave me the strength to endure until the end. Cancer is nothing to play with; it is a serious ailment. When something is serious and harmful, you must take serious measures to defeat it.

Chemotherapy and radiation treatments are no joke; however, you can and you must know that you can get through them. Yes, it all sounds pretty intimidating and scary when you hear it and have to go through it. Now, unless you are just going to give up and lay down and die, the treatments are do-able! If I did it, all of you who are going through it or will have to go through it in the future can make it. As the old song says, "You can make it if you try."

Now that I have gone through those two great challenges, I have a responsibility to share what I have experienced with others. I now view that whole experience as a test of faith. My test has become my testimony to the world that God is able to do exceedingly and abundantly more that you could ever think or imagine (Ephesians 3:30 KJV). Just remember that without faith in God, it is impossible to please Him (Hebrews11:6 NIV).

I write this book with much tenderness and understanding for those who are going through any form of cancer. I want to encourage you to keep the faith no matter what the diagnosis or prognosis may indicate. Always remember that there is another opinion that counts more than the rest, and that is God's final opinion. I continue to pray for a cure for this devastating disease, and I continue to keep cancer patients and their families in my daily prayers.

The Fear of Cancer Coming Back

One of the greatest fears that many cancer patients have is the fear of its return. The enemy, the Devil, wants to keep your mind in bondage in this way. Remember the Scripture that says God did not give you a spirit of fear but of power, love, and a sound mind (2 Timothy 1:7). Keep this Scripture close to your heart and allow God's spirit and His Word to keep your mind at rest. Rest in God! If your cancer comes back, also know that God is still with you just like He was the first time. He's not going to take you to the cancer battle without taking you *through it* once again.

Fear not, because God will be with you. Take a deep breath and get ready for the battle. We as thinking, intelligent individuals must not allow ourselves to be taken over by our thoughts. It is paramount when fighting against cancer to control your thoughts. Fear and doubt serve no good purpose, but they will drop you into such a deep depression that you will think you are dying when you are actually nowhere near death!

Thoughts about Suffering and Death

*M*any people do have a fear of dying, but if you can conquer that fear, then most of your battle is over. We must acknowledge that we are all born to die. No one will escape this process. The sooner we face this fact, the better off we will be. None of us knows the day or the hour of our departure, so why worry about it? Ask God to take away the fear of death so that you can focus on living a fuller life today. I have learned through my cancer ordeal that each day is a special gift from God and that we should be living every day as if it were our last.

Jesus himself says that "in this world you will have tribulations, but be of good courage for I have overcome the world" (John 16:33b). If Jesus, who is God, has overcome all of the tribulations of our wrongdoings, through His shed blood on the cross, then we also have the ability to overcome the struggles that are placed in our lives. This means that since we belong to Christ, we must pick up our cross daily and follow Him. These trials and difficult situations are stepping stones to learning, growing, and helping to make us better people in God. These situations are the things that God uses to mature us in our faith, trust, and obedience to Him.

Through these encounters, we begin to understand that these are the tests in life that build our character and validate our testimonies, and from these testimonies we begin to find personal ministries in helping other people. People who have been or who are going through what you have already successfully overcome will be placed in your path so that you may encourage and assist them in making it through. People would really rather see a good sermon than hear one. They need to see people practicing what they preach, in other words, acting upon what comes out of their mouths. The old saying that actions speak louder than words is certainly true and appropriate here.

Our true God-given mission in life is to help others. Sometimes it takes a person a whole lifetime to find out the reason God placed him or her on this planet, and that is that he or she is put on this wonderful earth to reach and touch the lives of other people in a positive way. They realize that God wants them to share their lives and testimonies of His love, grace, mercy, faithfulness, and goodness.

If we show compassion, concern, patience, and love, we are reflecting God's true image. As a cancer survivor, I do understand the moments of doubt when you don't think you'll pass the test (the situation or trial), but hang in there. These are the moments when your mind says one thing and your body says something entirely different. You feel like you are not going to pass your test because your body and mind are feeling weak and unresponsive. At these challenging moments we must find activities that help keep us positive and occupied.

A gratifying goal during these challenging times can be the act of serving others. Those of us who have accepted Jesus Christ as our personal Savior are to bring hope to those who have no hope, because Jesus is the hope of the world. Not only is He the hope of the world, but He is also the Light of the World! Remember earlier I talked about the light at the end of every difficult situation; well,

He is that light in all of our darkness! When things get dismal and dark, He is that light that is going to lead you out! Darkness has no place when light enters. I personally believe it is God's will and desire for you to be healed and your health restored. The question now becomes, "Do you want this for yourself?" Do you have the fortitude, determination, and will to press on through your situation with trust in your Creator, God? If you want this for yourself, then press on to complete your treatments so you can join me and millions of others in being a cancer survivor!

When the Battlefield Becomes Level Ground for All

I have noticed that regardless of race or economic status, people suffer and go through stressful situations in similar ways. I noticed as I struggled with my cancer experience that whether a patient was rich, poor, black, or white, and no matter how privileged one may have been, we were all the same when it came to the cancer treatments. We all tried to get through those experiences as quickly as possible. We began to encourage each other as the days passed. No one was exempt from experiencing the same treatments, symptoms, and side effects of the treatments. Cancer brings all cultures, ethnic groups, and social levels of people down to a common battlefield.

As we all counted down the days left for our treatments, we found we were all rooting for each other. When a person made the announcement they had completed their treatments, everyone celebrated and cheered! It made you feel good to know that other people going through the same situation were happy for you! It motivated all of us to continue with determination. Things like status, race, religion, and prosperity that sometimes separate people were no longer barriers because we were sharing in an experience that brought about community. Black, White, and Latino were all together talking and sharing our personal stories, as well as our cancer stories. There was no big *I* and little *you* as I saw it. We all encouraged each other to keep going and keep pressing on. We all looked forward to our day of freedom!

At some point in the journey, you realize you've come too far to give up! You start to understand you must focus on having a successful recovery. Have your cheering team on the sidelines urging you to keep going. By having your own cheering group, you set yourself up for victory and staying in the battle on the road to success.

Your success or failure is demonstrated by how you face the different fears and challenges that accompany cancer. Addressing those fears and challenges by calling upon the power of God and His Word helps you to keep them in check.

If fear is not allowed to control your emotions, then it has no effect on your mental state. This is how you want to slay all the little demons that accompany the cancer giant. When you are able to keep fear at bay, then you have conquered a great deal of the *scariness* of cancer. You will also find that it isn't as big as people make it out to be! In other words, cancer will not seem as fearsome as its reputation suggests. Now, I'm not trying to take anything away from cancer's devastating effects and lull you into a false sense of security, but I am saying don't let the word *cancer* put you in a place of paralyzing fear where you become stuck there. This is what you don't want.

From Testimony to Ministry

It now has been six years since my cancer diagnosis and treatment. I openly share my story with people facing cancer and other ailments. When windows of opportunity open, I am not ashamed to talk about my amazing faith journey. God has been too good to me for me to hold back my story. This book is another way to do just that. To get through your ordeal and not share your story to encourage other people going through the same fate is being totally ungrateful for how good God has been to you. Getting through the process is quite an accomplishment, but we must all admit that God played the biggest part in making sure this happened. I am not minimizing the expertise and importance of the cancer staff at the University of Chicago; however, I know that a loving God was the real miracle behind my recovery.

Established Cancer Support Groups

There are a myriad of cancer support groups available for cancer patients and cancer survivors. Most reputable hospitals will have cancer support groups. There are also cancer support groups in different communities, making it convenient for cancer patients to attend. If you have access to a computer, you can find anything you want pertaining to cancer on the Internet. Use these resources as opportunities for you to connect with others who are facing or have faced the journey of cancer. Let them be your support system and encouragement as you experience your journey.

Once you perform an Internet search, you will find there are many cancer groups that are more than willing to walk with you through your cancer journey. There are plenty of choices to meet your every need. I personally have not visited any support groups because of the large support system I already have. It appears that my new ministry is to walk with others going through the cancer process. I am praying now about starting up a cancer support group.

Fundraising Events

In 2006, the Y-Me Breast Cancer Mother's Day walk was able to raise $30 million in funds to donate toward finding a cure for breast cancer. I was a part of that endeavor. I walked with a strong desire to continue to contribute in any way I could to help raise funds to continue the work that is being done in breast cancer research. I believe that a cure is really close. I don't know why I feel this, but I do. I pray continually for a cure to be found, not just for breast cancer, but for all cancers. The different cancer walks and runs are doing a tremendous job at raising money. I will be participating in more of these walks to help the cause. If you have an interest in donating or participating in any of the events to raise money, then call your nearest cancer center to find out how you can assist them.

The Y-Me Breast Cancer Walk occurs every Mother's Day in downtown Chicago, but there are many other events that go on throughout the year in which you can participate. Your local hospital or cancer center has information on other fundraising events throughout the year. You can always telephone the American Cancer Society for their events too.

Walking with Other Women Diagnosed with Cancer

God allowed me to walk with women who had been diagnosed with different kinds of cancer. I have seen the uncertainty and frustration on their faces. I have been there to support them mentally. I encouraged each of them not to allow the enemy, Satan, to get control of their minds through paralyzing fear. Memorizing Scripture as I have suggested before is a powerful weapon against negative thoughts and fear. I encourage them to find some Scriptures that help to empower them mentally, spiritually, emotionally, and physically.

The women I have journeyed with are listening to and following the advice I have given them through my own experiences. I am able to share with them what kept me mentally tough throughout the situation. My advice to each woman is to trust God, His love for them, and His Word, which help to sustain them. Sometimes things don't always work out like we plan, but God knows about us and what we are going through. I tell them to remember God already has the plan worked out. We who are followers of Christ must keep our faith in Him without wavering.

Even when it doesn't look like our situation is improving and even when the doctor comes back with a bad report, we must at those very times cast our cares and burdens on God. When the burden becomes too big for us to carry, we must reach for that extra faith deep within us and say that "God is still in control of my situation" and quote those Scriptures that reaffirm what God says He will do in our situation.

You must build your mind up with those Scriptures that will help pull you through tough mental challenges. Hearing unpleasant reports from the doctor is challenging to anyone. However, if we know where our faith lies, we have the ability to reach deep within ourselves and know that God will take care of us. This is my advice to you. If you can just hold on to the fact that God is concerned about what you are concerned about and is with you through every situation, that will ease the pressure and the fear that the enemy tries to use to get you upset and scared.

If you can remember this, you'll be surprised at the strength you can develop. You'll begin to ask yourself, "What has come over me?" Trust me, I've been there. When my breast surgeon told me that he would have to reopen the incision he made from the first surgery, I was not pleased with that news, especially since the first incision was completely healed. It was a matter of concern that he reentered the incision to make sure he had gone far enough with the surgery, to what cancer surgeons call the *clear zones*. This means that all the areas around the malignant tumor have been removed to the clear areas of the breast where there is no malignancy. I had to ask God for strength to take me through another surgery, and He provided it!

The women that I spoke to and encouraged were at the beginning of the process, which means that they were at the point of having lots of tests. One woman was in the radiation and chemotherapy process. Some were going for second and third opinions. Wherever the women were in their process, they were all going through the same anxieties and concerns that I had experienced. At first you aren't sure just how to feel, so fear has its way of creeping into the situation when you're not even aware that it has. Sometimes you don't even realize that it is fear. In those moments when you're not sure just what is going on, that's when you must calm yourself, stop and take a deep breath, and readjust your mind and pray.

From Breast Cancer to Sharing God's Word

*A*s a breast cancer survivor, I believe that I now have to turn the page of breast cancer to think about what the experience has meant for me. As I turn the page from breast cancer, I have become keenly aware that the experience of having it has made me more sensitive to how important it is to live each day to the fullest. Life is precious and a gift from God. The cancer experience has helped to deepen my trust and faith in God.

I take away from this experience a wealth of knowledge and a better understanding of myself and of my faith. I have never taken the relationship that God has established with me for granted. I truly thank Him for allowing me to call Him my Savior, Father, Creator, and Lord. I count it a blessing that I found Him early in my life so that when trying times come, I feel His protection, guidance, counsel, and love. Cancer is a terrible disease that destroys every healthy cell of your body to which it is allowed to spread. I know that God was aware of its presence in my body even when my primary doctor wasn't.

He prepared me for the experience when I walked in the Y-Me Breast Cancer Walk in May 2006. It was this very experience that I reflect upon now and know that God was in the midst of my situation before I was even diagnosed with cancer. One of my colleagues in ministry helped me to understand that God was walking alongside me then. It's ironic to think how God does some things in such a way that you can't deny it was Him orchestrating the entire situation. Many times we take credit for how things turn out when it's really God's hand moving in it. His thoughts are truly higher than our thoughts and His ways higher than our ways (see Isaiah 55:8-9). We must stop and reflect upon every situation and give credit where credit is due. If we learn to do this, we will begin to see that the credit is due only to God.

As I turn the page of cancer, I pray that God will continue to keep my spirit, mind, and body healthy and strong. Living as a cancer survivor challenges me to forget what is behind and press on toward what is before me. I can't continue to look back at the most trying nine months of my life and relive those moments. I really don't care to anyway!

God has not brought me through the experience so that I can constantly have a pity party over the experience, but He has brought me through because I still have a work to do for Him. I now find myself walking through the cancer experience with others who are learning how to slay the cancer giant through the Word of God. The Scriptures tell us that God's Word is a lamp unto our feet and a light unto our path (Psalms 119:105). If this is true, why aren't we using His Word to light our path? The path may be through the valley of cancer, but there is a light that leads the way, if we will only follow it!

As I turn the page of cancer, I also want to leave an encouraging word to those of you who are just beginning your journey, are in the middle of your journey, or ending your journey. The message of encouragement I want to leave with you, wherever you are in the journey, is that God is with you, no matter how stressing your situation may seem. He is with you and He cares about what you are going through because He loves you. You must hang on to the fact that He is right there in the struggle with you. It's truly like the footprints in the sand, where at the end of the journey you only see one set of footprints because He's been carrying you most of the way!

Allow the love of God to enter your body and your mind. You may be wondering how that can happen. This is how it happens. Find a comfortable chair, preferably a recliner so your feet are elevated, sit back, close your eyes. Try to erase everything from your mind, take a deep breath and then slowly feel the Spirit of God that lies within each of us to minister to you. Meditate on the things of God, His Word, and the vastness of His love.

This type of love is almost beyond comprehension. It is even more extraordinary because God Himself is that love! A person must once in his or her lifetime stop and think how truly awesome God is. We have to think about His omnipotence (his power), His omnipresence (he's everywhere at the same time), and His omniscience (he knows all things). Psalm 139:4 (NLT) even says that God knows what you're going to say before you say it. Now tell me if God is not worthy of all our trust!

The only way we can even begin to thank this awesome God for our salvation is to serve him. I don't know of any person who would be willing to send their only child to a place where that child would face an ungodly death. I can't help but think how I would feel if I had to send my own son to his death in order to save the world! Let me stop and pray, "God, help me to remember your great sacrifice of your son so that my son and others might be saved. Never let me forget the price your son paid for us on Calvary." The gift that each Christian received as a result of His son's death is beyond understanding. I don't even know if "thank you" is an appropriate expression of gratitude for what God did for us. There are no words adequate to express appreciation for experiencing that kind of love.

When we think about this in the light of our cancer journey, we must ask ourselves how far God would go to save us from the devastation of cancer. Well, He has already shown us through the death of Christ. He is love, so we know He loves us individually. Since He is omnipresent; He is with us at all times. He is omniscient; therefore He knows everything, including what we are thinking and feeling. He also knows that our minds can be weighed down with the possible effects of cancer.

However, because He is with you, you don't have to worry about your circumstance because He is working it out in the spiritual realm. Because He is omnipotent, all powerful, and still in the miracle-working business, believe that your situation can change for the better in the twinkling of an eye or even while you are on your knees praying. That's how awesome and wonderful God is. So, my sister or brother, put your faith in God and trust Him to see you through. Don't give up; keep pressing forward with the Word and the love of God hidden in your heart.

Afterthoughts about My Battle with Cancer

It's very easy after you have successfully gone through your cancer surgery and treatments to have thoughts about your mortality. It's inevitable if you are a thinking human being. When we walk through the valley of the shadow of death, we face death with its cold, ugly face and have thoughts of dying. We don't quite know how to feel when doctors and others say we are cancer free. Because we are human and thinking beings, we ask ourselves, "Am I really?" This is when we could possibly begin to weigh ourselves down with unnecessary secondary thoughts and worries.

This is where we must learn to take one day at a time in the land of the living. With God's help we must continue to keep control over our mind and thoughts. As a cancer survivor, I'm working on training myself with God's help to think positive, healthy, and spiritual thoughts. We must learn to overcome thoughts of our cancer returning and any other negative thoughts. This in itself is helping you to defeat the cancer giant. Worrying and wondering if your cancer is going to come back only throws your body into a stressful state, which promotes the conditions for cancer cells to survive. Let's keep those cells dead!

Myths Concerning Breast Cancer

There is so much misinformation about breast cancer that it warrants some warnings to the reader. Breast cancer does not just strike middle-aged and senior women and men. It affects all age groups, from the young woman in her twenties to the senior women in their sixties and seventies. Don't be uneducated about the facts on breast cancer. Breast cancer can strike women who have had no family history of the disease. It can strike women who are perfectly fit, as well as those who are unfortunately unfit.

Breast cancer cannot be contracted from someone else. It is not passed sexually. If you have the cancer gene, it doesn't necessarily mean you will get cancer. Breast cancer can be treated successfully. Women aren't the only ones who can carry the cancer gene. Men do as well—even though they might not have the disease, they can pass on the gene. There are many more myths about cancer, so make yourself aware of them so that you will have a proper understanding.

I knew that breast cancer was in my family history, and I wasn't completely oblivious to the fact that it could happen. However, I couldn't believe it would happen at the time that it did. It just stunned me how it struck at the most unpredictable time ever. I had to get healthy to find out I was unhealthy. It was truly an oxymoron! That's just it—you can't know when some misfortune will happen to you, but you can be aware and educated to the facts and realities of the health conditions in your family background. Don't let myths about this deadly disease keep you in denial. Learn all you can about family ailments and be knowledgeable.

A Word of Encouragement and Hope

My desire is for the readers of this book to be encouraged and filled with hope by the strengthening of your minds with the Word of God. It is my prayer that you will begin and continue your journey with God as you battle the demon of cancer or any other devastating problem. Cancer is a demon with giant-sized terror, but be aware that terror weakens us spiritually through our minds. It can do this only if we allow our minds to be overpowered by the lies that cancer tries to evoke in us. It takes a strong mind and trust in God to fight and slay the giant of cancer.

Some individuals will allow the forces of depression and despair to wreak havoc with their spirit and weigh them down physically. Now we must rely on the doctor's expertise to help us fight off the devastating effects of the disease itself, but that's only 50 percent of the battle. The other 50 percent is a transformed and renewed mind in Christ Jesus. Now there may be some of you who say this is all kind of far-fetched. My reply to you is that I have lived through the cancer battle and I have been there. I fought the good fight of faith in God by drawing upon His Word to empower me mentally and, in many instances, physically.

It was the love I felt from God, His power, the reading of His Word (the Bible), excellent doctors, and my faith in God that brought me through a fierce battle with cancer. I could feel the presence of an all-powerful God surrounding me and sustaining me. I constantly prayed that His will would be done. He says to "ask me and I will tell you some remarkable secrets about what is going to happen here" (Jeremiah 33:3 NLT). We must be like Jonah when he was deep in the belly of the whale and cried out to God for help. I found myself calling out constantly for God to be with me as I journeyed through the whole cancer experience. Thank God He answers those who call upon His name.

Scriptures that Bring You Strength

In this section of the book, I will suggest some Scriptures in the Bible that will empower you as you go through your journey with cancer. Please take some time to meditate on these Scriptures so that you can become familiar with them. I hope that these Scriptures motivate you to search the Bible for yourself in order to build mental strength against the negative thoughts that like to creep in when you are not expecting them. Remember, I have suggested that the best way you can fight mentally against cancer and slay the negative thoughts it provokes is to saturate yourself with the powerful Word of God. I really can't stress this enough, and that's why you see it so many times in this book.

Fortify your thinking with the Word! Now, some of you might think that I am talking about the Bible too much. Well, I will not apologize for this. I'm only telling you what I learned as I fought off the defeating and unproductive thoughts that cancer brings. I am an ordained minister of the gospel of Jesus Christ, and my charge is to spread the good news of the Word of God. I take an enthusiastic position on the Bible because I believe it to be true, and as Paul states in Romans 1:16 (NIV), "I am not ashamed of the gospel of Christ, because it is the power of God for the salvation of everyone who believes, first for the Jew, then for the Gentile."

I truly believe in Jesus, the Son of God, who died for my sins over two thousand years ago. I am glad that God, His Father, decided to send Him into this world in human flesh to save me from my sins. I understand that without Him coming to this earth as a human to redeem me back to God, I would be on my way to hell! That's why I am honoring God with this book, to help others be reconciled to God. This is my way of saying, "Thank you, Lord, that you have adopted me into your family and all the rights and privileges that you offer your children are mine."

I am also writing this book to encourage people who are going through situations like serious illness, depression, unemployment, loss of a loved one, or any other traumatic and unexpected circumstance that life throws at you. I want you to know that God is the same yesterday, today, and forever, and He will see you through whatever it is you are experiencing. Trust and faith are the two things that move God to work on your behalf. Trust that He is working on your situation. Have faith that He will help you to get through it, and not only will He help you get through it, but He will take you through it!

When you are hurting, God is also hurting. What concerns you also concerns God. We as God's creation must learn to call upon God in every situation, whether it is good or bad. In Isaiah 33:11, it tells us to call upon Him and He will answer. Stop, right now, allowing our adversary, the Devil, to steal your peace of mind. Take back what he constantly tries to steal from each of us. Demolish unhealthy and unproductive thoughts of death and defeat. Reject the kind of thinking that says that there is nothing you can do about your situation. The Devil is a liar! The Scriptures say that Satan is the father of lies. Now, do you want to believe anything that a liar whispers in your ear? I don't think so, because I think you are smart enough to know that when a person tells one lie, he must tell another. One lie always leads to another. No one that I know wants to hang around a liar, because a liar always causes trouble and *is* trouble. Don't let the Devil lie to you and tell you that you'll never get over what you're going through. We don't have to accept that because we have a guaranteed hope, which is in Christ Jesus.

Keep looking up to Jesus. To help you do this, start by reading and meditating on the following Scriptures:

> Isaiah 41:13 (NIV) "I am the Lord, your God, who takes hold of your right hand and says to you, 'Do not fear; I will help you.'"

> Psalm 103:2-3 (KJV) "Bless the Lord, O my soul, and forget not all his benefits: Who forgiveth all thine iniquities; who healeth all thy diseases."

> Exodus 23:25 (AKJV) "I will take sickness from the midst of thee."

> Proverbs 4:20-22 (KJV) "My son, attend to my words; incline thine ear unto my sayings. Let them not depart from thine eyes; keep them in the midst of thine heart. For they are life unto those that find them, and health to all their flesh."

> Matthew 8:17(NLT) "This fulfilled the Word of the Lord through Isaiah, who said, 'He took our sicknesses and removed our diseases.'"

> Isaiah 53:5(KJV) "But he was wounded for our transgressions, he was bruised for our iniquities: the

chastisement of our peace was upon him; and with his stripes we are healed."

Matthew 9:35(KJV) "And Jesus went about all the cities and villages, teaching in their synagogues, and preaching the gospel of the kingdom, and healing every sickness and every disease among the people."

Matthew 10:1(NLT) "Jesus called his twelve disciples to him and gave them authority to cast out evil spirits and to heal every kind of disease and illness."

Matthew 12:15 (KJV) "But when Jesus knew it he withdrew himself from there; and great multitudes followed him, and he healed them all."

Matthew 14:14 (KJV) "And Jesus went forth, and saw a great multitude, and was moved with compassion toward them, and he healed their sick."

Luke 6:17-19 (KJV) "And he came down with them, and stood in the plain, and the company of his disciples, and a great multitude of people, out of all Judea and Jerusalem, and from the seacoast to Tyre and Sidon, who came out to hear him and to be healed of their diseases; And they that were vexed with unclean spirits; and they were healed. And the whole multitude sought to touch him: for there went virtue out of him, and He healed them all."

These are just a few Scriptures to get you started in searching God's Word for yourself to find verses that will encourage and empower you to think about being healed and delivered from your situation. If He was going about healing two thousand years ago, He is still doing the same today. As many of these scriptures point out, Jesus was not selective in His healings. All who were sick and brought to Him were healed. He demonstrated His healing power, then He empowered and encouraged His disciples to do the same. Make no mistake; God wants everyone to be healed, otherwise He would not have had His son suffer on the cross for that cause. Someone might say, "Well, if that's true, how come I'm still sick?" For that person I first suggest that you go to God and ask God why you are suffering so. God always has the answer. Secondly, I suggest that you ask yourself these questions: Do I have a problem trusting God to deliver me? Am I having a pity party about my situation? Do I have a faith level problem in believing that God is in control? Do I lose myself in defeating thoughts rather than go to the Word of God for comforting and empowering thoughts? Do I like the attention that I receive from others as an ill person? When have I sought the Bible for strength and encouragement? Do I even own a Bible? Do I know that the Bible has the answers to most of life's questions? Have I kept God in His rightful place in my life since I started this ordeal? Yes, self-examination of where you are spiritually, emotionally, and mentally with God is a step that will catapult you into the reality of your situation. It will also help you to understand your relationship with God.

You will realize that you either have a close and intimate relationship with God, or you may painfully find that you have a fragmented or nonexistent relationship with God. If you find yourself in the latter situation, God is waiting with open arms for you right now to ask Him into your life. Quickly ask for His forgiveness, repent of the sins that are keeping you out of fellowship with Him, and ask Him to come and live in your heart. Correcting a fragmented or nonexistent relationship with God is that simple! We all place God on the back burner of our lives. We make major decisions without Him. We don't call on Him in prayer when we're facing serious situations. We don't spend daily quality time with Him through the reading of His Word (Bible), praying to Him, or listening to Him.

Then we find ourselves facing cancer or some other serious situation, and we don't know where to turn, or whom to trust, or where to put our faith. We somehow get amnesia. Shame on us! Remember the song I mentioned earlier called, "Jesus Is on the Mainline," which tells us to call Him up and tell Him what you want! Yes, we forget about the one who can do all things. Not only can He do all things, but He can do the impossible! How could we forget someone like that? It's beyond my comprehension.

Living as a Cancer Survivor

As a cancer survivor, I sometimes am not sure just how I feel. Most of the people that I've heard who proudly announce that they are cancer survivors do not display the same feelings I have. Usually, I'm more perplexed than anything else. I'm perplexed because I still have questions in my mind about why some people survive cancer and others don't. I don't want to second-guess God, but it is mind boggling that I survived cancer, yet a good friend of mine passed away from it! This question might not ever be answered on this side of life, but hopefully I will understand when I get to the other side and stand face-to-face before God.

Don't mistake what I am saying. I do thank God for His omniscience, omnipotence, and omnipresence and for sustaining my life. However, my finite mind can't always comprehend the way He does things. Life truly is in His hands, and we as ordinary individuals won't always understand the workings of God. The only thing we can do in difficult situations is to just believe and have faith that God knows what He is doing. We must pray and ask God to help us to understand in our hearts that He does know the end from the beginning! Again I say, I have learned to take one day at a time and thank God for each and every day that I remain among the living.

Life as a cancer survivor puts a great deal of pressure on me personally to be an advocate of early detection. Early detection increases chances of surviving. I believe my charge now as a cancer survivor is to encourage women and men to get yearly examinations and help them to understand that they must take charge of their health. When you have God, a loving and supportive family, good friends, your right mind, and your health, you have everything. Living as a cancer survivor allows me to influence people to be more aware of how it can quietly develop while you're feeling just fine and least expect it. I believe God has kept me here for a reason, and I know part of the reason is to walk with others who are facing cancer. Since I have come through it successfully and believe that I am completely healed, I must continue on my own journey to help others believe they can get through cancer too.

Supporting Cancer Research

I spent the second Sunday in May in 2006 and 2007 walking in the Mother's Day Walk in downtown Chicago. I used the event in those years to honor and to remember my mother, who succumbed to breast cancer, and friends who have died of cancer, as well as to reflect on my own personal experience with cancer. It helps me to keep in perspective the responsibility I have of raising women's awareness of the destructive and devastating effects of cancer. I am committed to sharing my experience with as many people as possible. Raising funds is the very least I can do to help find a cure for this disease and honor those who have lost their lives fighting it.

I walked to raise funds because I believe in the value of the research being done. I walked to raise funds because I have reaped the benefits of the research. I walked to raise funds because there is still much work remaining to find cures and discoveries to be made that will one day eradicate cancer entirely.

When I reflect on my bout with cancer and how well I was taken care of during my treatments, the availability of the chemotherapy and radiation, and the expertise of a team of professionals who planned and carried out my treatment, I am grateful to God for the progress that has already been made. Many individuals and organizations have been giving generously to help fund the continuous research to find medicines that fight the disease. Those of you who are reading this book and are interested in seeing cancer eradicated can help by making a financial donation to the American Cancer Society.

Advancements in the Treatment of the Cancer Giant

I am truly grateful for the advancements that have been made in the last twenty-six years since my mother died of cancer. The availability of treatment and the progress made in treatments have been transformative. Now women have a much greater chance of beating cancer and living longer. My mother did not have the quality of treatment that professionals are able to provide now. Since I was her main caregiver, I was able to see her form of treatment and now I'm able to compare her treatment with mine.

The difference between my mom's treatment and mine is the advancements that have been made in the kinds of chemotherapies and radiation treatments available. Also, I believe the way chemotherapy and radiation treatments are administered today versus the way they were administered twenty-six years ago is more specific and individualized. They are given more in line with the individual needs of the patient. For instance, my mother always received her chemotherapy intravenously and I had mine given to me through a process called the PUSH system, which I mentioned earlier. My chemotherapy sessions lasted approximately ten minutes, while my mother's lasted approximately three hours! Whatever your procedure, make sure it is the very best for you. Talk to your doctors and don't be afraid to ask questions. Expect to get your questions answered.

The biggest advice I would like to leave with you is to read and educate yourself with all the information you can find about your specific cancer. Also go online and get information about the doctors who will be treating you. Find out what their area of expertise is. Find out their reputations and their history of success.

Learn about cancer procedures and treatments. Don't leave it up to the doctors to provide all the information you'll need. Have someone with you who can take notes on what the doctors are telling you, because you won't remember all that is said to you. If you have someone taking notes, you can review them when you need them. I personally found this to be extremely helpful. Be smart and informed. Look up terms that doctors use to describe your illness. Have a good medical dictionary at your disposal. These are just a few suggestions that might make your journey a little more bearable. Read and search out answers for yourself. Don't let your mind deceive you into thinking that the less you know, the better off you are. This is a trick of Satan!

Since I started this book, I have revealed to my oncologist that my family on my mother's side had a high incidence of breast cancer. When I informed her of this, she suggested that I have the BRCA tests done to see if I carried the cancer gene. It was confirmed through testing that I do have the BRCA gene. With that finding, I was then able to talk with my son about his health and medical options. In sharing this information, he will be well informed and able to make intelligent health decisions.

This information is invaluable when you have had a family history of breast cancer. Thus, I encourage all women who have a high incidence of breast cancer on both sides of your family to take the BRCA test to find out if you have the gene. Be aware that if you have the cancer gene that you must also be vigilant about having your ovaries checked because you are more prone to get ovarian cancer as well! If you have the cancer gene, your children also need to be tested to see if the gene was passed on to them. This is the proactive attitude that I spoke of earlier. Always try to be on top of your situation!

Other relatives in your family, both close and distant, who share a common bloodline, should be made aware of the possibilities of having the BRCA gene. This information can be a valuable aid in early detection. I am now trying to find some relatives in upper New York from the Sherman Brown family who need to get this information. I am speaking of Sherman Brown who was once married to Mary Billingslea, and they had a daughter whose name was Gladys. If you are reading this book and you know of this family, please pass along this information.

Well-Meaning People after the Journey

*I*t is understandable that people who care about you or know of your cancer journey will try to inform you of statistics and the latest findings in cancer research, but the continuous bombardment of that kind of information, after your treatment is completed, can be disheartening. I know they are trying to show their sincere concern by doing this, but for me it is very difficult.

They send articles, cards, and e-mails giving you statistics on nutrition, and a myriad of do's and don'ts for the cancer survivor. I can speak for myself by saying I know that people think they are helping to keep you informed, but I have found that sometimes the information that they send you is not true. For instance, I have gotten many e-mails saying that cancer feeds on sugar. This is not a correct statement. I spoke to my oncologist and a nutritionist who both said this is absolutely untrue. That's why it's critical that you become educated about your particular cancer and what needs to be done to keep your body healthy and cancer free.

My oncologist encouraged me to continue to follow a low-fat diet and continue to exercise so that I might continue to remain cancer free. This in itself is motivation for me to do what is nutritionally correct. Exercise is the main factor in keeping my weight down and being able to stay healthy. I have always been pretty active throughout my life, so I just have to continue to be consistent in my efforts. My eating habits were not the worst, yet not the best before I had cancer. I have, however, become more cognizant of the food I eat. I am more aware of the variety, quantity, and quality of foods I eat.

I have cut down on my portions and I eat smaller meals throughout the day. I make a concerted effort to stay away from sugary and fatty foods. I don't drink beverages with caffeine or drinks containing high levels of sugar. I make great efforts not to eat carbohydrates that lack nutrition (those made with white flour). I have cut down tremendously on fried foods and foods containing saturated fats.

I know that people think they're helping you stay abreast of the facts, but sometimes they can be a hindrance by constantly reminding you of your journey with cancer. You want to function as a healthy, healed person, not one who is constantly reminded of the difficult bout you had with cancer. How you handle these well-meaning people is totally up to you.

The television is another medium that constantly bombards you with facts on cancer or is constantly making you aware of who has had a recurrence of cancer. Don't get discouraged, because each person's journey is totally different. Not all women have had a recurrence of breast cancer. Acknowledge in your spirit, heart, mind, and soul that you're not going to have a recurrence of cancer, and live your life every day with this mindset. Believe that God has healed you and keep your trust in Him. Don't let what other people deposit in your spirit, especially if it is negative, remain in your spirit or your subconscious mind. Rid yourself of those thoughts and stay positive no matter what.

Live each day for that day. Don't worry about what's going to happen tomorrow, next week or even next year. Live for the moment you're in! Don't put off for tomorrow what you can make happen for today. Stop and take time to smell the roses. Listen to the birds sing their songs. Notice the beauty of the sky. Spend time with people who mean the most to you. Do the things that make you happy and keep you motivated and positive. Don't spend time thinking about negative thoughts and discouraging comments said to you by other people.

~~~

Some Reflections from My Main Supporters

*M*y book wouldn't be complete if I didn't share some reflections from the people who were with me throughout my entire ordeal with cancer. So I decided to pose a question to three people who ventured with me through my cancer journey. I asked my husband, my girlfriend, and my son the following question concerning their feelings as they cared for me throughout my cancer therapy. The question was as follows, "What was the most difficult period for you during my bout with cancer?" I asked each of them to answer this question and give their comments about the journey. The following chapters contain their comments, and my personal messages to other supporters.

The Long Wait (My Husband's Reflections)

I talked to my husband, Willie, concerning this question. This is what he had to say to me. The first words he uttered were, "The long wait." I didn't understand right away what he meant, so I asked him to elaborate. He went on to say that all the events that had already transpired, meaning surgery, chemotherapy, and radiation, didn't bother him as much as the one-year wait for the doctor's recovery prognosis after the completion of the therapy process. He considered *that* the longest and most difficult period for him during my cancer experience. He wanted all the doctors' assurances that, after the one-year period, all would be well with me. Of course, it was impossible for them to be completely sure that this would be the case! He said that with all I had gone through, he personally needed to believe and to know that I was alright. He ended by saying, "Seeing you go through the debilitating effects of chemotherapy and radiation, and not being able to do anything to help, was also difficult."

I understood then that he realized the situation was something he had absolutely no control over, and both of us had to totally trust God and the expertise of the doctors. I know it was as scary for him as it was for me when I was given the first chemotherapy and radiation treatments. Even though it was over quickly, neither of us knew just what my reactions would be. Thank God I really had no negative effects at that point! I can say most of the treatments went pretty much the same as the first. The day of the treatment, I was fine. It was the *day after* shot that took me down, with fatigue and nausea!

A Message to My Husband

To Willie, my husband of forty-four years, I say thank you for journeying with me through numerous health challenges. You have been by my side through them all. I know my bout with breast cancer placed a great deal of stress on you, emotionally, spiritually, and financially, but you have never faltered. You were my strength in this nine month battle. It was your attentiveness and care that helped me to endure this ordeal and I will never forget all that you did. I still remember how you cared for me forty-two years ago when I was challenged with health issues early in our marriage. You were my pillar of strength then and you remain my pillar of strength now. You have a very generous and kind heart, and that is why God continues to bless your life. He blesses you because you bless others. I have gained wisdom from being married to you. I pray that God blesses us with many more healthy years together! I love you very much.

Moving Forward (Thoughts from My Girlfriend)

When I asked my constant companion and friend, Gloria, how she felt as she journeyed with me through my bout with cancer, she said she felt helpless as she watched me go through the process, but she also recognized that my spiritual being was getting stronger, which caused me to press forward with trust and faith in God. I imagine this must have been quite encouraging to her. At least, I hope so. Watching her encourage me as I went through the process was a little difficult for me because I knew she was trying to be strong for me. She did finally confide in me that she had cried when she first received the news that I had cancer. I can imagine it was pretty tough for her.

I can't really put into words the support and encouragement I received from Glo, as her friends call her. She is a very amazing woman of faith. She is serious about her walk with Christ. Just seeing her during those nine months of tribulation helped me keep going. She always had a smile, a prayer, a word of encouragement, and a devotional to share. She helped me keep my eye on the future. Even though she never spoke about my sickness, she did feel sometimes when I was making very serious decisions that I needed to take more time to think about my options. She shared these thoughts after the process. She was concerned that sometimes I might have acted too fast. However, I felt that too much time had already been wasted with getting the wrong diagnosis from my primary doctor at that time. I do know that sometimes haste makes waste, but in this case, I felt I needed to act quickly.

I knew that Gloria would back any decision I made, even if she didn't always agree. I love her for her continuous support, love, and concern. She really encouraged me when she told me that she had never seen a day during my therapy treatments that I had not made myself presentable. I believe she was telling me in her own way that she was proud of me! Gloria, how can I say thanks for the many things you did for me and with me when I was going through one of the most stressful times in my entire life? As I said, words cannot express the love, concern, and support that you gave to me. All I can say is, "I love you," and I will always be there for you when you need me. I will always be just a telephone call away. I will always be your sister in Christ!

At this point I also want to give a special thanks to Reese, Gloria's husband, for allowing Gloria to spend so much time with me during the whole process. I never felt he resented the time that Gloria spent with me. Reese, I want to thank you for being so understanding and sensitive to my needs. I did need a friend to walk with me and hold my hand through one of the most difficult times of my life. I know you sacrificed precious time with your wife. I want you to know that I appreciate your generosity! You never complained when Gloria left the house early to pick me up for a therapy session and returned late in the afternoon or near evening! Thank you, thank you, thank you.

A Message to My Friend

Gloria, I believe you already know that you are a very special woman. I know you know that I am one of your biggest cheerleaders. You have touched the lives of so many people that it makes it easy for me to tell you the impact you had upon me as I fought breast cancer. Your personality and wonderful smile are so powerful that they would light up anyone's life. Many times your smile was the lift I needed to press on. Your attentiveness and faithfulness made me want to fight the fight and to pass the test I was struggling against. Your words encouraged me to keep the faith, and your actions let me know that you wanted me to succeed. I know it was a personal sacrifice for you to accompany me to every appointment I had, but you did it for nine months! Thank you, thank you, thank you! You are a gem of a friend. I treasure our friendship, and this I think you know. You were a constant companion when I really needed one. I will never forget how you were there for me. Please know that you will always hold a special place in my heart. My wish for you is that God will continue to use you as His instrument of love and as the powerful preacher of His Word that you are.

Is She Really Okay? (My Son's Thoughts)

When I talked with my son, Tony, he told me his greatest concern came when he would ask how I was doing as I was going through my treatments. I always said I was doing fine. Because my response was always the same, he wondered whether I was telling him the truth! He said as long as I was okay, he was okay. However, he often wondered if I was really going to be okay. Tony just needed to be sure all was really well with me. I imagine it had to be very devastating for him as an only child to hear that his mother had cancer. It had to be pretty unnerving, but he did a good job of hiding it!

I assured him that I had told him the truth. I was really okay during the whole ordeal. I told him that I wasn't fearful, sad, or worried about getting well because from the beginning, I placed my trust and faith in God. In other words, I was saying to my son that I placed myself and my confidence in the hands of Almighty God. My purpose for telling him this was to emphasize the point that I allowed God to be God. All I did was to stretch out on faith. To quote Hebrews 11:1 once again seems appropriate: "Now faith is the substance of things hoped for and the evidence of things not seen."

My hope and trust was in God. I also trusted the team of doctors that God had led me to. I hope my ordeal with cancer will be a testimony to you that without God we can do nothing, but with God all things are possible.

I know how I felt when I heard that *my* mother had cancer. It was one of the scariest moments in my entire life. Being an only child myself, I couldn't imagine not having my mother with me. So I prayed and I prayed that she would get well, but that didn't happen. I did find out, however, that life does go on, even if you feel you have lost the most important person in your life. Tony, life does go on. Make good use of the time you have here on earth. Life doesn't always go the way you want it to go, so just make sure you keep your hands in the hand of God. Take care of your family, and all of you keep moving forward with God.

A Message to My Son

Tony, this is a personal message from me to you. I know that since you were a young child I have tried to introduce you to the Christian faith and the Lord Jesus Christ. I might not have totally succeeded, but I did the best I knew how. However, now that you are grown, I want to take this opportunity to stress to you how important it is to live for God. The blessings and the prayers that He has already answered for you should be evidence and testimony enough for you to know that God is awesome. He is loving, compassionate, and kind. All He asks of us is that we get to know Him on a personal level by studying His Word.

I want you to know that daily devotion (time with God) is a must. Why, you might ask? Well, time with God is life sustaining. Spending time with God before you start your day guarantees that He will be with you throughout your day. Now, this may sound simplistic to you, but take it from one who has been in this world a lot longer than you. Life really has no meaning without God. He is the only someone who can change the course of your life for the better. Can you just take my word for it? Because I love you, I would not steer you wrong. I only want what is best for you, Simone, and Chogie.

I couldn't have faced cancer the way I did if I hadn't had the security of knowing that God first, your father second, and great doctors were taking care of me. I was grateful I allowed God and only God to take charge of my situation. I rested in the comfort of that fact. Trust me, that fact alone allowed me to focus on getting well. Son, I want you to know Jesus like that. Take time to become intimately knowledgeable about Him. The reason He died for you was so that you would love and serve Him. Find a church you can belong to and become active in, and then watch how your life will change. If you think things are going well now, just watch how much favor God will personally bestow upon you and your household. God bless you and your family as you worship, pray, and seek God together! Always remember the old adage, "A family that prays together stays together!" It's true, son, it's true. Train your daughter up in the fear (reverence) and the admonition of the Lord. May God bless you and your family. I send lots of hugs and kisses to you, Simone, and Chogie.

A Message to All of My Other Friends

I want to convey here a big *thank you* to all of my other friends who took the time to encourage me during my fight against cancer. The telephone calls and the visits from persons near and far meant the world to me. I cannot tell all of you who prayed for me, waited on me, e-mailed encouraging expressions to me, came and sat with me, cleaned and cooked for me how appreciative I was of all of your kindnesses. I will never be able to express in words or repay you for your concern, caring spirits, and your presence while I was unable to care for myself. It takes special kinds of people, Christian people, who strive to serve God through serving others to show the concern and care you gave to me. A very special *thank you* is written to my very good friends, the Kanes and their family in Maryland and my Aunt Carolyn in Florida. My wish for all of you is that you are blessed exceedingly and abundantly above all that you could ask or think, according to the power that works in you (Ephesians 3:20).

A Message to the Breast Cancer Team at the University of Chicago

A person does not really understand the importance of having good professional medical care until she or he is stricken with serious illness. When you are unable to take care of yourself and have to depend on others, you are very vulnerable and to some degree helpless in your situation. The bedside manner of medical professionals can encourage you or discourage you, depending on each doctor or staff member. When you have a doctor who is sincere, listens to you, and shows understanding of your concerns, you can consider yourself blessed. This was the case when I arrived at the University of Chicago Hospital. I was put at ease the moment I arrived at the Breast Cancer Center by a wonderful young lady who greeted and attended to me with great enthusiasm and a warm smile. Her gentle nature and the way she approached me caused me to take a deep breath and relax.

As I continued in the care of the University Hospital, I encountered many people who had the same wonderful effect on me. This included my cancer team, which I mentioned earlier in the book. I cannot say enough concerning the doctors, staff, and other people I met during my treatments and chemotherapy sessions at this wonderful hospital. My message to this great team and breast cancer center is that you make people feel that you care about their lives when they walk into your great facility. I don't think I exaggerate when I say that you make your hospital an awesome place to come when a person is sick. I would recommend your hospital to anyone who is searching like I was for a place where they can feel affirmed, listened to, and supported.

I refer many people to your hospital when they are looking for someplace to have their medical needs addressed. I want to say *thank you* for your professionalism, your empathic spirit, and finally for your continued work throughout your hospital. I thank the doctors, the cancer staff, the people in the Breast Cancer Center, and those people working in the cancer radiology department. May God continue to bless your work as you continue to find cures and answers to the devastating illnesses that are ravishing and killing people in our communities all over this nation and the world.

A Message to the Emmaus Community

Lastly, I could not complete this book without remembering to thank the Emmaus Community for their serious concern and fervent prayer for me as I travailed through my cancer treatments. I want to thank the pastors of this church community for making me feel like I was important and I was missed. On a number of occasions they conference-called me to have prayer as I was about to leave for chemotherapy, and their timing was always perfect. I cannot tell you how much those calls meant to me! There is no greater encouragement to a person when she is sick than to hear from or see her pastor or, in my case, my pastors. Their prayers gave me the strength to face the day. When you have a faith community to support you in tough times, you find strength and comfort in their visits and words. Other people from this community sent words and cards home to me while I was recuperating. Some came and visited with me. Others called. I really felt special and blessed, all at the same time. It was wonderful to learn how I had touched the lives of others through ministry. Many people expressed this to me when I returned to worship. I think my recovery was due to my determination to get back to worship so I could praise God for His faithfulness in my situation. I wanted to assemble with the people I worshiped with as soon as possible so that I could begin to feel normal again. When I was able to do this, I never looked back! It was the medicine I needed to really get me going again. Thank you for your many expressions of love. My prayer is that God will bless the pastors and the entire Emmaus Community beyond measure. I also want to thank the pastors for allowing me to work with them in ministry.

My Final Thoughts

It was very gratifying for me to reserve a section of this book to thank all of the people who supported and journeyed with me through my bout with the cancer giant and who gave me the courage I needed to slay the terror of this giant. It was quite a battle, but I fought the good fight of faith and defeated this foe. I now write this book as a survivor and memorial for all of the women in my family who succumbed to this devastating disease. I am convinced that my struggle and survival will end a long family history of women dying from breast cancer. The progress and discoveries that cancer researchers are using now to treat breast cancer have won and are winning this battle for many women today. I can only continue to pray that someone will find the cure for all cancers. I believe that the cure for cancer is just around the corner. With the medical strides that researchers and doctors are making, it wouldn't surprise me to hear the announcement that a cure has been found in the not-so-distant future! This is what I will be praying for, so that people will no longer have to suffer from this debilitating and insidious disease.

Since I have one more preventive step left for me to remain cancer free, I'm writing this book to remind myself and you of how good and wonderful God has been. I have remained cancer free until this very day, since my surgeries and therapy six years ago, even though I carry the cancer gene. God is truly amazing, and He is still healing His people from sickness and disease.

Epilogue—My Message to the Readers

My reason for writing this book was to encourage, enlighten, introduce, or reintroduce people suffering from serious illness to our loving and compassionate God. The intent of this book was to share my own personal bout with the serious illness of cancer and give some insight as to how I personally took control of my situation with the help of God. I wanted to really emphasize how people have the option of giving in to the difficult situations that they find themselves in or taking control of each situation, no matter how threatening it might be. You can be unproductively reactive or productively proactive. The choice is ultimately yours.

This book is written to encourage you to be assured in any situation that God is with you because He loves you and cares what happens to you. In any situation you face, you are never alone. He never leaves you. All you need to do is trust, have faith, and believe that He wants the very best for you. Although illness will befall many of us, we can overcome it if we keep our trust in God. Keep a positive mental, spiritual, and emotional attitude, and watch God work in your situation. Give God praise even before you see the manifestation of your healing.

God bless you for reading this book. My prayer is that it has brought you comfort and helpful information and moved you to have a closer walk with God. I mainly wanted to say to you to take care of yourself. If I have done this, then I thank God for impressing upon me to attempt this endeavor. One of Martin Luther King Jr.'s favorite sayings is from an old song, "If I can help somebody as I pass along, then my living will not be in vain." This describes my sentiment also and the very reason I wrote this book!

Written Resources Used in this Book

Unless otherwise indicated, Bible quotations are taken from *Today's Parallel Bible*, which contains the following:

New International Version, Zondervan Publishers, Grand Rapids, MI, Copyright, 1973, 1978, 1984, International Bible Society.

New American Standard Bible, Zondervan Publishers, Grand Rapids, MI, Copyright, 1960, by Lockman Foundation, A Corporation Not for Profit, La Habra, CA.

Updated Edition of the King James Version

New Living Translation Version, Published by Zondervan Publishing House, Grand Rapids, MI 49530, Copyright, 2000.

The Message, Eugene H. Peterson, New Testament with Psalms and Proverbs, NavPress Publishing Group, P.O. Box 35001, Colorado Springs, CO 80953, Copyright, 1993, 1994, 1995.

www.ingramcontent.com/pod-product-compliance
Lightning Source LLC
Chambersburg PA
CBHW020436290526
45785CB00002B/878